KANISHKA SINGH
ANSHUMAN JAMDADE
SATYAPAL YADAV

# PHARMACOTHERAPY FOR TOBACCO CESSATION

KANISHKA SINGH
ANSHUMAN JAMDADE
SATYAPAL YADAV

# PHARMACOTHERAPY FOR TOBACCO CESSATION

## Pharmacological Aids in Tobacco Cessation: Mechanisms and Efficacy

LAP LAMBERT Academic Publishing

Cover image: www.ingimage.com

Publisher:
LAP LAMBERT Academic Publishing
is a trademark of
Dodo Books Indian Ocean Ltd. and OmniScriptum S.R.L publishing group

120 High Road, East Finchley, London, N2 9ED, United Kingdom
Str. Armeneasca 28/1, office 1, Chisinau MD-2012, Republic of Moldova, Europe
Managing Directors: Ieva Konstantinova, Victoria Ursu
info@omniscriptum.com

Printed at: see last page
**ISBN: 978-620-8-44247-7**

# PHARMACOTHERAPY FOR TOBACCO CESSATION

**Author**

**Dr. Kanishka Singh**

**Co-Author**

**Dr. Anshuman Jamdade (BDS, MDS)**
**Professor & Head of Department**
**Oral Medicine & Radiology**

**Dr. Satyapal Yadav (BDS, MDS)**
**Professor**
**Oral Medicine & Radiology**

**Dr.Neeraj Kumar (BDS, MDS)**
**Professor**
**Oral Medicine & Radiology**

**Dr. Amrita Aggarwal (BDS, MDS)**
**Reader**
**Oral Medicine & Radiology**

# ACKNOWLEDGEMENT

This Research work was possible only because of great efforts put by large number of people. It would leave avoid in this dissertation, if their efforts are not acknowledged.

First of all, I would like to thank the Almighty god for giving me a good life.
I am eternally obliged to lot of kind individuals who have helped me whole heartedly during every step of this research work and have reaffirmed my faith in human nature. I am very grateful to my grandparents **Late Sh. Arjun Singh & Smt. Raghuviri Singh** for their unconditional love and blessings, my parents **Dr.Pushpendra Pal Singh & Mrs. Urmila Singh**, for their patience and support and making me what I am today. Without their support, I would not be able to purse my post-graduation. At the very onset I would like to convey my heartful gratitude to my parents who have been the backbone in every aspect of my life. I especially owe thanks to my younger brother **Mr.Aayushman Singh** who has been a constant source of love and energy through all these days. I am incredibly grateful to my cherished in-laws **Mr. Harveer Singh & Mrs. Ramrati** and my husband **Dr. Shivam Chahar** for their unwavering support, encouragement and understanding during the journey of completing this research work.

As I grapple with feelings of resentment, I find myself at a loss for words to adequately convey the depth of gratitude, indebtedness, and appreciation I harbour towards **Dr. Anshuman Jamdade**, my esteemed guide, distinguished educator, erudite scholar, and exemplary mentor in the realm of Oral Medicine and Radiology. Their profound expertise has profoundly influenced the trajectory and substance of my research endeavours. I am sincerely thankful for their unwavering patience, empathetic support, and relentless encouragement that have accompanied me every step of this transformative journey. I am fortunate to be under his unlimited source of knowledge, skill and the perfection he desires in his work and sees in his students.

Words are too meagre to express my heartfelt gratitude towards my Co-guide **Dr. Satyapal Yadav,** Professor. I am truly fortunate to be under his unlimited source of knowledge, skill and perfection. I am more than indebted for his unsurpassable guidance, benevolent attitude and giving me a sense of professional duty. Their presence, understanding and belief in me have been a constant source of strength and inspiration.

I express my deepest gratitude to **Dr.Neeraj Yadav** (Reader), **Dr. Amrita Aggarwal** (Reader) for their expert opinion, motivation and support during the preparation of this study and throughout my post graduate course.

I would like to post my sincere thanks to my colleague **Dr Monika Gupta**, **Dr Saurabh Kanawa** for being a greatest support & helping hand throughout. I immensely thanks to my seniors **Dr. Falaknaz Khan, Dr.Anuja Sharma** and **Dr Kanupriya Sharma** and my junior **Dr. Reeya Garg** for their constant care, support and stood by me whenever I needed them the most.

I would like to post my heartful thanks to **Dr Himanshi Kumawat** for all the advice and wise words he has provided me over the time being.

In the end I wish to thank all those who have directly and indirectly contributed to the completion of this dissertation.

**Dr.Kanishka Singh**

## CONTENTS

# INTRODUCTION

Tobacco refers to the plant species Nicotiana tabacum, which is cultivated for its leaves, which are dried and processed for various uses, particularly smoking, chewing, or snuffing. The primary active ingredient in tobacco is nicotine, a highly addictive substance. Nicotin causes Relaxation during stress, Improved attention, learning, reaction time and problem solving; Reduced hunger etc. Tobacco products come in various forms, including cigarettes, cigars, pipe tobacco, chewing tobacco, and snuff. Tobacco is used in various ways, which include smoking forms as (Beedis, Cigarettes, Cigar, Cheerot, Chhutta, Dhumti, Hookli, Hookah, Chillum, Pipe), smokeless forms (Pan, Pan masala, Mawa, Khaini, Mainpuri tobacco, Chewing tobacco, Snuff), tobacco products for application (Mishri, Gul, Lal dantmanjan, Bajjar, Gudakhu, Creamy snuff, Areca nut preparation (Areca nut, Supari, Meetha mawa). In India, Beedi is most popular form of tobacco smoking followed by cigarette smoking. Pan with tobacco is major form of chewing tobacco[1].India is the second largest consumer of tobacco in the world. The prevalence of tobacco use among men hasbeen reported to be high in most parts of the country (generally exceeding 50%). Its use is more common in rural areas as compared to urban areas[2].

Smoking has numerous immediate health effects on the brain and on the respiratory, cardiovascular, gastrointestinal, immune and metabolic systems. Tobacco use causes a wide range of major diseases which impact nearly every organ of the body. Tobacco-related illnesses such as cancer and cardiovascular and respiratory diseases are already major problems. Tobacco use is a risk factor for six of the eight leading causes of death in theworld. Smoking tobacco causes cancer of the lung, larynx, kidney, bladder, stomach, colon, oral cavity and oesophagus as well as leukemia, chronic bronchitis, chronic obstructive pulmonary disease, ischemic heart disease, stroke, miscarriage and premature birth, birth defects and infertility, among other diseases.Tobacco use also causes economic harm to families and countries due to lost wages, reduced productivity and increased health-care costs.[3] By the year 2020, tobacco will become the world's largest single health problem, causing an estimated 8.4 million deaths annually, claiming more lives than HIV,tuberculosis, maternal mortality, motor vehicle accidents, suicide, and homicide, combined. Deaths in developed regions are expected to rise nearly 50%, from 1.6 million to 2.4 million, while deaths in Asia will soar almost four-fold from 1.1 million in 1990 to an estimated 4.2 million in the year 2020.[4] By the end of this century,tobacco may kill a billion people.[3] Tobacco use has economic implications for the society and nation as a whole. Individual household's economic implications of tobacco include direct cost of tobacco products and indirect cost due to the expenditure arising from the adverse health effects of tobacco use.

There are many ways (pharmacological and non- pharmacological) in which the menace of tobacco can be countered and diminished if there is a political will and collective societal commitment to strengthen tobacco control. Tobacco dependence treatments are effective across a broad range of populations. Numerous effective medications are available for tobacco dependence, and clinicians should encourage their use by all patients attempting to quit smoking.[5] The purpose of this library dissertation is to provide available knowledge on various pharmacological interventions currently available and its Indian scenario.

# OBJECTIVES

The aim of this Library Dissertation is to comprehensively evaluate and summarize the effectiveness, safety, and practical application of various pharmacological interventions in helping individuals quit smoking or using tobacco products.

# REVIEW OF LITERATURE

## TYPES OF TOBACCO[6]

## SMOKELESS TOBACCO

Smokeless tobacco is usually consumed orally or nasally, without burning or combustion. There are two main types of smokeless tobacco: snuff and chewing tobacco.

1. **DRY SNUFF**- Dry snuff is powdered tobacco that is inhaled through the nose and absorbed through the nasal mucosa or taken orally. Once widespread, particularly in Europe, the use of dry snuff is in decline.
   - Most Prevalent:Europe

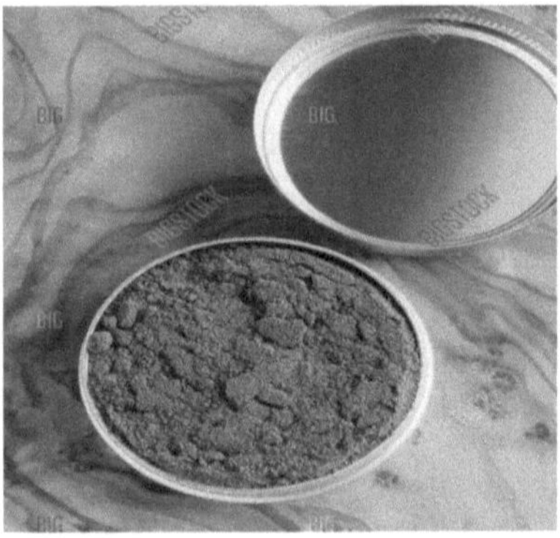

2. **MOIST SNUFF** - Moist snuff is a small amount of ground tobacco held in the mouth between the cheek and gum. Manufacturers are increasingly pre packaging moist snuff into small paper or cloth packets to make the product more convenient. Other moist snuff products are known as khaini, snus, shammaah, nass, or naswa.
   - Most Prevalent: Worldwide

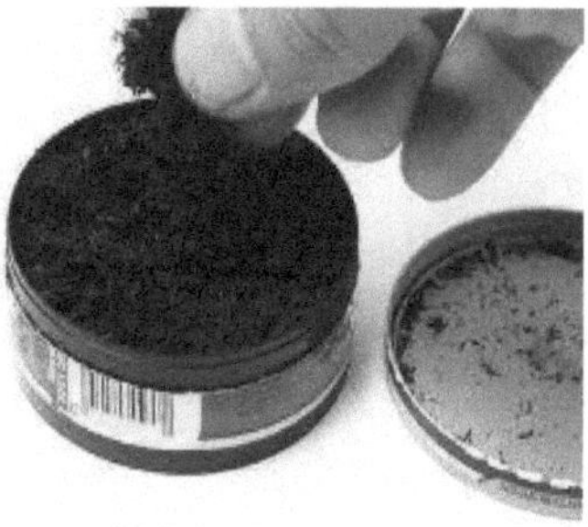

3. **CHEWING TOBACCO** - Oral smokeless tobacco products are placed in the mouth, cheek, or inner lip and sucked (dipped) or chewed. Tobacco pastes or powders are similarly used, placed on the gums or teeth. Sometimes referred to as "spit tobacco" because users spit out the built-up tobacco juices and saliva, this mode of tobacco consumption became associated with American baseball players during the twentieth century. The tobacco industry exploited these sports heroes to market their tobacco products to youth. Smokeless tobacco causes cancer in humans and leads to nicotine addiction similar to that produced by cigarette smoking. There are many varieties of smokeless tobacco, including plug, loose-leaf, chimo, toombak, gutkha, and twist. Pan masala or betel quid consists of tobacco, areca nuts (Areca catechu), slaked lime (calcium hydroxide), sweeteners, and flavoring agents wrapped in a betel leaf (Piper betel). There are endless varieties of pan masala, including kaddipudi, hogesoppu, gundi, kadapam, zarda, pattiwala, kiwam, and mishri.

- Most Prevalent: India

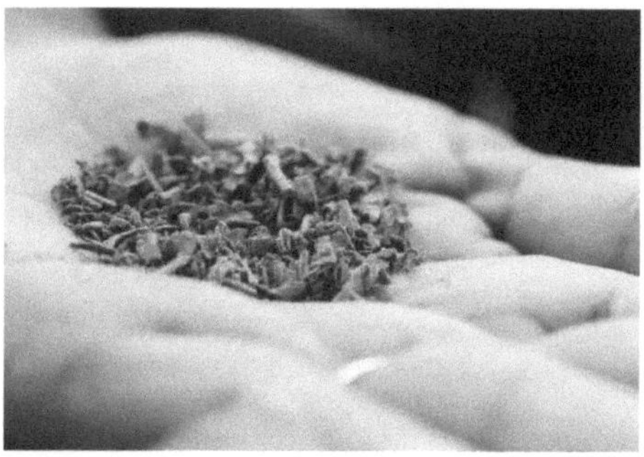

## SMOKING TOBACCO

Tobacco smoking is the act of burning dried or cured leaves of the tobacco plant and inhaling the smoke. Combustion releases biochemically active compounds in tobacco, such as nicotine and TSNA, and allows them to be absorbed through the lungs.

1. **ROLL-YOUR-OWN (RYO)**-cigarettes are cigarettes hand-filled by the smoker from fine-cut, loose tobacco rolled in a cigarette paper. RYO cigarette smokers are exposed to high concentrations of tobacco particulates, tar, nicotine, and tobacco-specific nitrosamines (TSNAs), and are at increased risk for developing cancers of the mouth, pharynx, larynx, lung, and esophagus.

- Most Prevalent: Europeand New Zealand

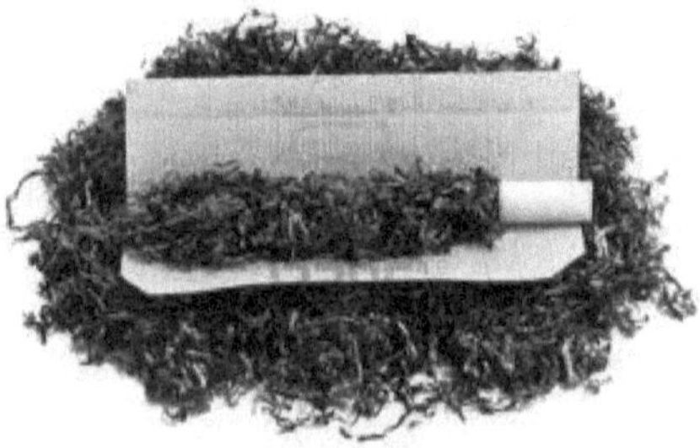

2. **MANUFACTURED CIGARETTES** - are the most commonly consumed tobacco products worldwide. They consist of shredded or reconstituted tobacco, processed with hundreds of chemicals and rolled into a paper-wrapped cylinder. Usually tipped with a cellulose acetate filter, they are lit at one end and inhaled through the other.

- Most Prevalent: Worldwide

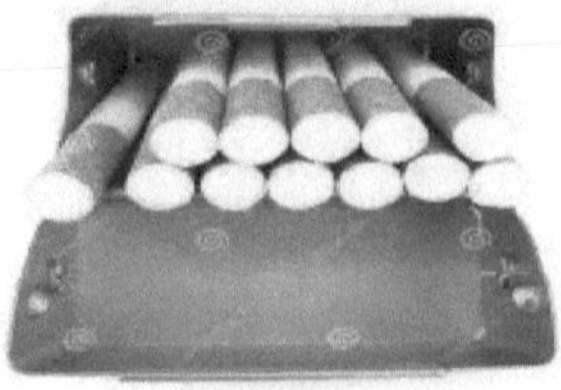

3. **CIGARS-** Cigars are made of air-cured and fermented tobaccos with a tobacco-leaf wrapper. The long aging and fermentation process produces high concentrations of carcinogenic compounds that are released on combustion.The concentrations of toxins and irritants in cigars are higher than in cigarettes. Cigars come in many shapes and sizes, from cigarette-sized cigarillos to double coronas, cheroots, stumpen, chuttas, and dhumtis. In reverse chutta and dhumti smoking, the ignited end of the cigar is placed inside the mouth.

- Most Prevalent: Worldwide

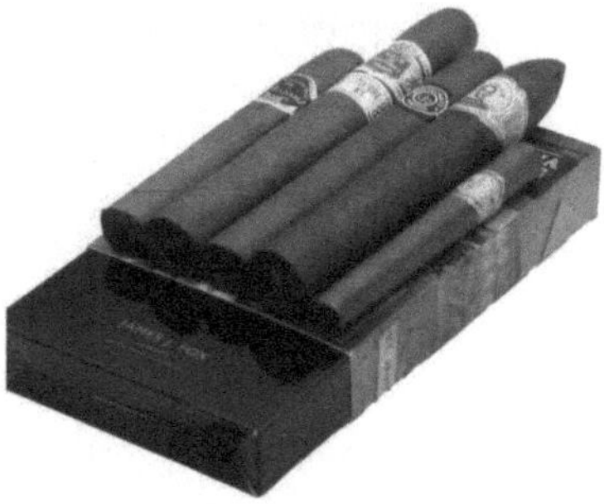

4. **BIDIS-** consist of a small amount of sun-dried, flaked tobacco handwrapped in dried temburni or tendu leaf (Diospyros sp.) and tied with string. Despite their small size, bidis deliver more tar and carbon monoxide than manufactured cigarettes because users are forced to puff harder to keep bidis lit. Bidis are found throughout South Asia and are the most heavily consumed smoked tobacco products in India.

- Most Prevalent: SouthAsia

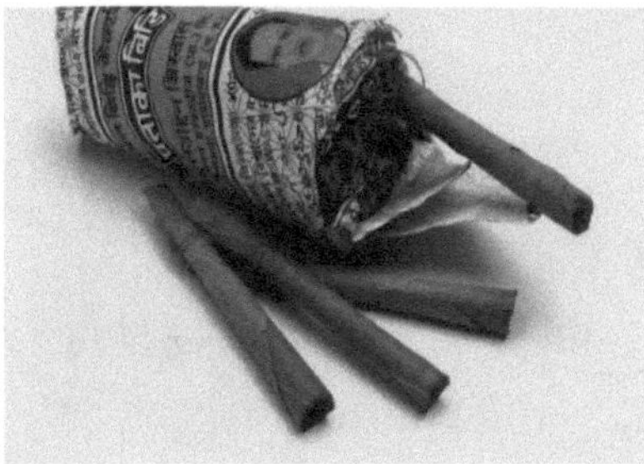

5. **KRETEKS** - Kreteks are clove-flavored cigarettes widely smoked in Indonesia. They may contain a wide range of exotic flavorings and eugenol, which has an anesthetic effect, allowing for deeper and more harmful smoke inhalation.

- Most Prevalent: Indonesia

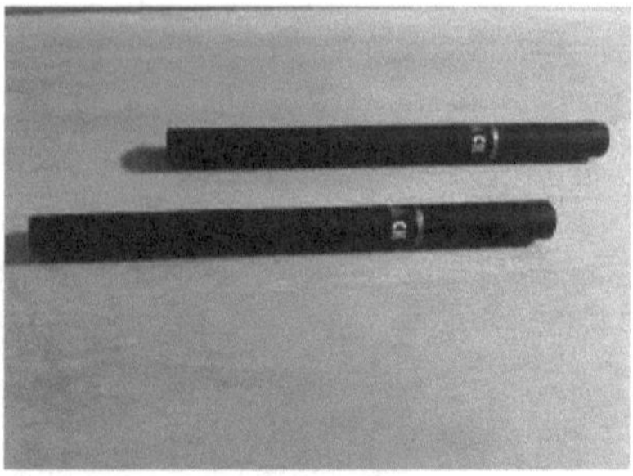

6. **WATER PIPES** -Water pipes, also known as shisha, hookah, narghile, or hubble-bubble, operate by water filtration and indirect heat. Flavored tobacco is burned in a smoking bowl covered with foil and coal. The smoke is cooled by filtration through a basin of water and consumed through a hose and mouthpiece.

- Most Prevalent: North Africa, the Mediterranean region, and parts of Asia

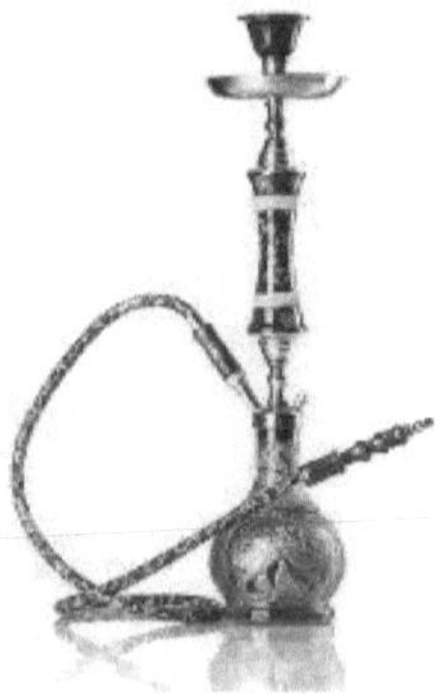

7. **PIPES** - Pipes are made of briar, slate, clay, or other substances. Tobacco is placed in the bowl, and the smoke is inhaled through the stem. In Southeast Asia, clay pipes known as sulpa, chillum, and hookli are widely used.

- Most Prevalent: Worldwide

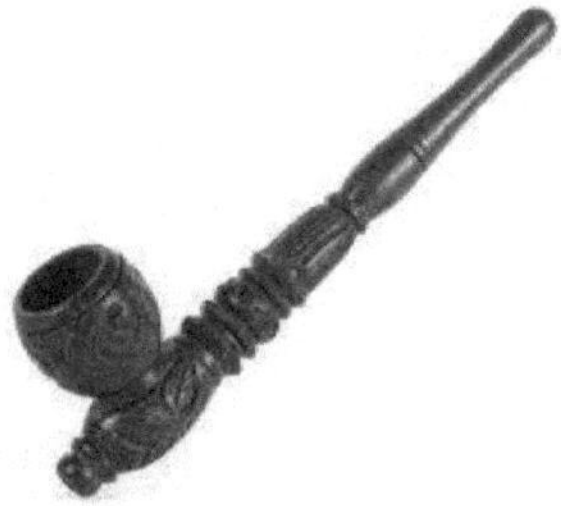

8. **STICKS** - Sticks are made from sun-cured tobacco and wrapped in cigarette paper—for example, hand-rolled brus.

- Most Prevalent: Papua New Guinea

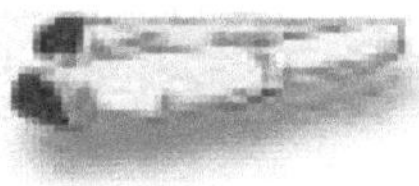

# HARMFUL EFFECTS OF TOBACCO

## EFFECTS OF SMOKELESS TOBACCO[7]

Smokeless Tobacco and Cancer

- Many smokeless tobacco products contain cancer-causing chemicals.
    - The most harmful chemicals are tobacco-specific nitrosamines, which form during the growing, curing, fermenting, and aging of tobacco. The amount of these chemicals varies by product.
    - The higher the levels of these chemicals,the greater the risk for cancer.
    - Other chemicals found in tobacco can also cause cancer. These include:
        - A radioactive element(polonium-210)found in tobacco fertilizer
        - Chemicals formed when tobacco is cured with heat (polynuclear aromatic hydrocarbons—also known as polycyclic aromatic hydrocarbons)
        - Harmful metals (arsenic, beryllium, cadmium, chromium, cobalt, lead, nickel, mercury)

- Smokeless tobacco causes cancer of the mouth, esophagus, and pancreas.

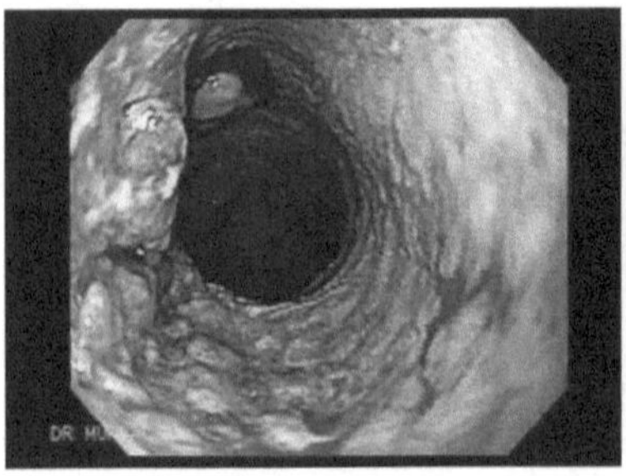

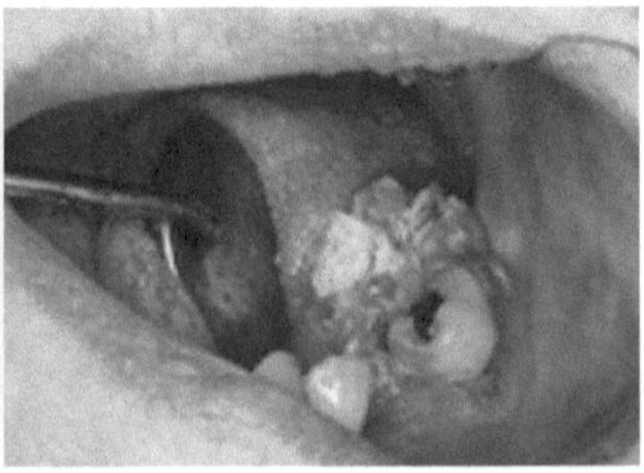

Esophagus cancer

Oral cancer

Smokeless Tobacco and Oral Disease

- Smokeless tobacco can cause white or gray patches inside the mouth (leukoplakia) that can lead to cancer.

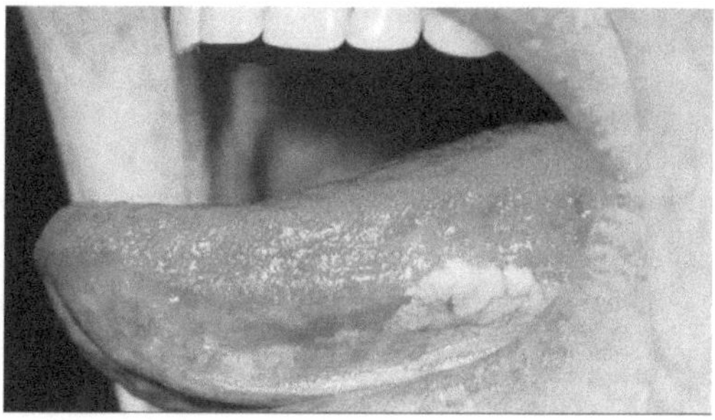

Leukoplakia of Tongue

- Smokeless tobacco can cause gum disease, tooth decay, and tooth loss.

Reproductive and Developmental Risks

- Using smokeless tobacco during pregnancy can increase the risk for early delivery and stillbirth.
- Nicotine in smokeless tobacco products that are used during pregnancy can affect how a baby's brain develops before birth.

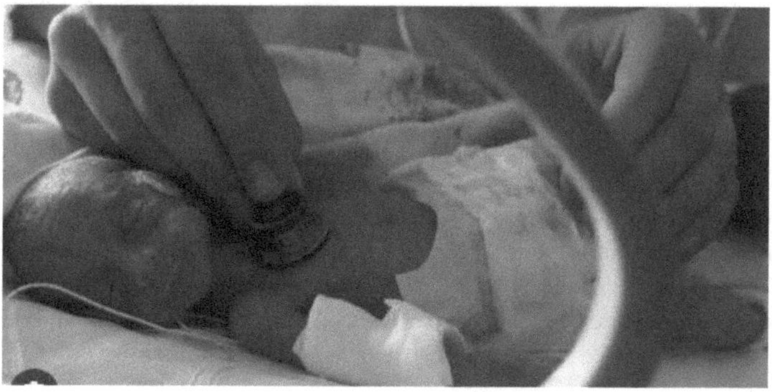

Other Risks

- Using smokeless tobacco increases the risk for death from heart disease and stroke.
- Smokeless tobacco can cause nicotine poisoning in children.
- Additional research is needed to examine long-term effects of newer smokeless tobacco products, such as dissolvables and U.S. snus.

## SMOKE TOBACCO[8]

Smoking and Increased Health Risks

Smokers are more likely than non smokers to develop heart disease, stroke, and lung cancer. Estimates show smoking increases the risk: For coronary heart disease by 2 to 4 times For stroke by 2 to 4 times Of men developing lung cancer by 25 times Of women developing lung cancer by 25.7 times Smoking causes diminished overall health, increased absenteeism from work, and increased health care utilization and cost.

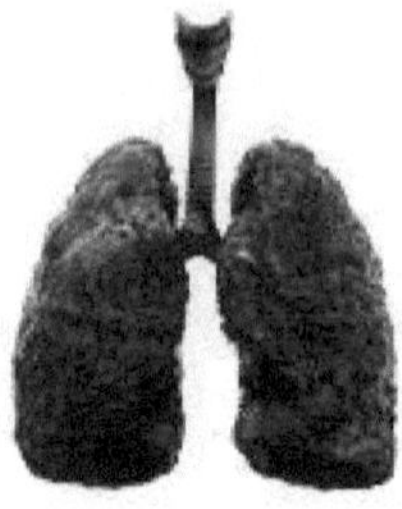

Lung cancer

Smoking and Cardiovascular Disease

Smokers are at greater risk for diseases that affect the heart and blood vessels (cardiovascular disease). Smoking causes stroke and coronary heart disease, which are among the leading causes of death in the United States. Even people who smoke fewer than five cigarettes a day can have early signs of cardiovascular disease. Smokingdamages blood vessels and can make them thicken and grow narrower. This makes your heart beat faster and your blood pressure go up. Clots can also form. A stroke occurswhen: A clot blocks the blood flow to part of your brain; A blood vessel in or around your brain bursts. Blockages caused by smoking can also reduce blood flow to your legs and skin.

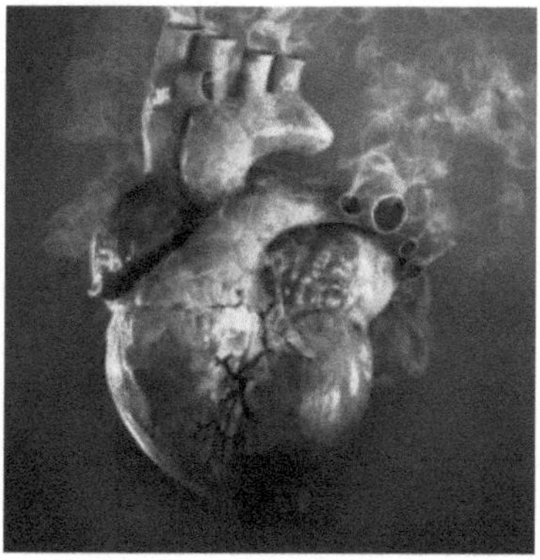

Smoking and Respiratory Disease

Smoking can cause lung disease by damaging your airways and the small airsacs (alveoli) found in your lungs. Lung diseases caused by smoking include COPD, which includes emphysema and chronic bronchitis. Cigarette smoking causes most cases of lung cancer. If you have asthma, tobacco smoke can trigger an attack or make an attack worse. Smokers are 12 to 13 times more likely to die from COPD than nonsmokers.

Smoking and Cancer

Smoking can cause cancer almost anywhere in your body: Bladder Blood (acute myeloid leukemia) Cervix Colon and rectum (colorectal) Esophagus Kidney and ureter Larynx Liver Oropharynx (includes parts of the throat, tongue, soft palate, and the tonsils) Pancreas Stomach Trachea, bronchus, and lung Smoking also increases the risk of dying from cancer and other diseases in cancer patients and survivors. If nobody smoked, one of every three cancer deaths in the United States would not happen.

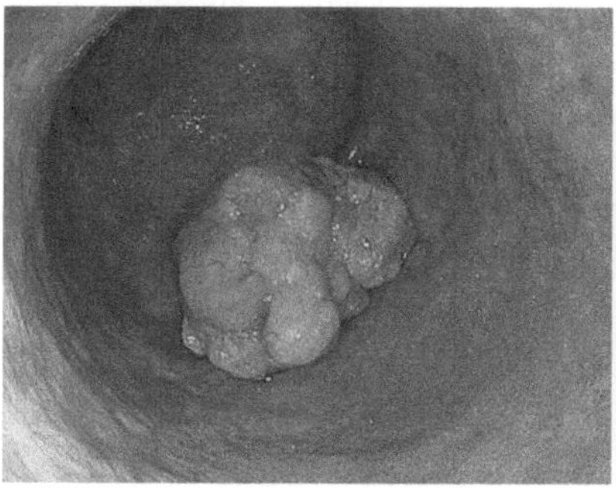

Stomach Cancer

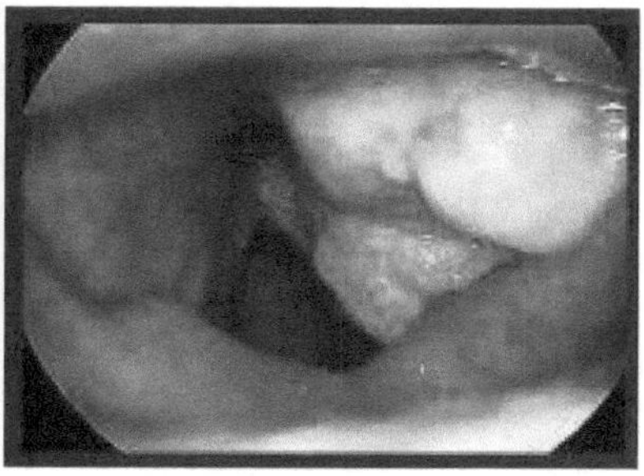

Laryngeal Cancer

Smoking and Other Health Risks

Smoking harms nearly every organ of the body and affects a person's overall health. Smoking can make it harder for a woman to be come pregnant. It can also affect her baby's health before and after birth. Smoking increases risks for:

- Preterm (early) delivery
- Stillbirth (death of the baby before birth)
- Lowbirth weight
- Sudden infant death syndrome (known as SIDS or crib death)
- Ectopic pregnancy
- Orofacial clefts in infants
- Smoking can also affect men's sperm, which can reduce fertility and also increase risks for birth defects and miscarriage.
- Smoking can affect bone health.

- Women past child bearing years who smoke have weaker bones than women who never smoked. They are also at greater risk for broken bones.

Smoking affects the health of your teeth and gums and can cause tooth loss.

Smoking can increase your risk for cataracts (clouding of the eye's lens that makes it hard for you to see). It can also cause age-related macular degeneration (AMD). AMD is damage to a small spot near the center of the retina, the part of the eye needed for central vision.

Smoking is a cause of type 2 diabetes mellitus and can make it harder to control. The risk of developing diabetes is 30– 40% higher for active smokers than nonsmokers.

Smoking causes general adverse effects on the body, including inflammation and decreased immune function.

Smoking is a cause of rheumatoid arthritis.

## 3.3 METHODS OF TOBACCO CESSATION

There are two types of interventions, namely non-pharmacological and pharmacological. Non-pharmacological interventions are important as they are cost effective such as Counselling by medical practitioners, Smoking cessation strategies delivered by nurses and support organizations, Telephonic call back and follow-up, health education and heavy taxation on tobacco products. When they are combinedwith pharmacological interventions, give better abstinence rates, even in resistant cases with frequent relapses. Various effective pharmaco-therapeutic methods for tobacco cessation are now available and should be advised to the tobacco abusers. Pharmacotherapy should be strongly recommended to all persons with severe dependence, tobacco users with multiple failed self-attempts, tobacco users unable to abstain with brief intervention alone.

- **Approaches for tobacco cessation at the individual level may be divided into 2 types-**

1. **Non Pharmacologic intervention:-**It includes

A) **Behavioural interventions:** A variety of behaviour therapies, ranging in complexity from simple advice offered by a physician or other health care providers or much more extensive therapy offered by counsellors, have been shown to be efficacious for tobacco cessation. The Five A's (Ask, Advise, Assess, Assist and Arrange) and Five R's (Relevance, Risk, Rewards, Repetitions, Roadblocks) arefive to fifteen minute research based counseling approach that has proven global success.[9]

B) **Telephone counseling:** The effectiveness of telephone counseling in aiding smoking cessation has been well-documented, particularly through the protocol developed by the American Cancer Society (ACS). This protocol, implemented since 2000, has significantly increased the success rates of sustained quitting, particularly among younger smokers. Despite its success, there is room for improvement in terms of cost efficiency.[10]

2. **Pharmacologic interventions:** Various effective pharmacological methods of smoking cessation are available which can help a person to quit smoking.[9]

## ➢ BROAD APPROACHES TO PHARMACOTHERAPY

**❖ Pharmacotherapy should be strongly recommended to[11]**

- All persons with severe dependence.
- Tobacco users with multiple failed self-attempts.
- Tobacco users unable to abstain with brief intervention alone.

- It may be suggested to all persons with lower levels of dependence who feel the need for some external help. For this group, lower doses of pharmacotherapy may be effective.

- However, it is important to note that "no form of pharmacotherapy is a substitute for motivation".

**❖ When to recommend pharmacotherapy?[11]**

If available, it must be strongly recommended to tobacco users with severe dependence which can be determined by any of the clinical indicators below:

- Using tobacco within the first 30 minutes of waking up. or
- Using more than 20 cigarettes or *bidis* everyday or using very high doses of smokeless tobacco.
- A score of more than 6 on the Fagerstrom questionnaire.

**❖ The choice of pharmacotherapy would depend on[11]**

- Any contraindications or precautions for use.
- The tobacco user's preference.
- Cost of the treatment (particularly where the cost is out-of-pocket).
- The clinicians' experience with recommending and supervising the pharmacotherapy.
- Generally, pharmacotherapy is advised for 3 to 4 months. However, some studies suggest using pharmacotherapy for longer periods of up to six months or more.

- ❖ **Type of treatment Rationale**[11]

✓ ***Nicotine replacement therapy***

-Supplies the nicotine but eliminates other (harmful) chemicals in the tobacco product.

- Decreases the intensity of cravings and withdrawal symptoms, enabling people to function better while dealing with the social and psychological aspects of their dependence.

- May provide some of the effects for which the tobacco user used the particular tobacco product (e.g. the desired mood or immediate support to cope with stress).

- Evidence-based pharmacotherapies currently available for nicotine dependence include the following:

Nicotine replacement treatments

- Gums
- Patches
- Sprays
- Inhalers
- Lozenges
- Sublingual tablets
- Silver acetate

✓ ***Non-nicotine replacement treatments***

- Act on central brain receptors and minimize withdrawal from nicotine when the tobacco user suddenly stops use.

Non-nicotine pharmacotherapy:

- Bupropion
- Varenicline

Other (clonidine, nortryptiline)

## NICOTINE REPLACEMENT THERAPY

Nicotine replacement therapies (NRTs) are smoking cessation medicines that release small amounts of nicotine into the bloodstream to help counter cravings and reduce other physical withdrawal symptoms. NRTs are used to slowly wean the smoker off of nicotine. The NRT products contain nicotine, which is equally addictive, but the NRT medications deliver smaller amounts of nicotine than cigarettes and without many of the other harmful effects of tar and carbon monoxide found in cigarettes. Additionally, NRT allows focusing on overcoming the psychological and behavioural aspects of smoking without the added difficulties of withdrawal symptoms. By reducing the symptoms of withdrawal, NRT can double an individual's chances of quitting successfully.[5]

Nicotine replacement therapies increase the rate of long-term quitting by 50%–70%. NRT users were twice as likely to remain off tobacco compared to NRT non-users four years after treatment. All forms of NRT appear to be as equally effective.[9]

**N L Benowitz and P Jacob (1990)**- A study was designed to test the hypothesis that i.v. replacement of nicotine will suppress daily intake of nicotine from cigarette smoking and to compare the physiological effects of prolonged exposure to nicotine infused i.v. to the effect of smoking cigarettes throughout the day. Eight subjects received a 14-hr infusion of deuterium-labelled nicotine dosed to achieve levels of nicotine similar to those while smoking cigarettes for each individual (average, 33.1 mg; range, 17.7-49.9 mg) or saline (placebo). Cigarette smoking was permitted as desired. Nicotine infusion did not significantly affect the number of cigarettes smoked or the amount of tobacco burned, but nicotine intake from cigarette smoking was suppressed in all but one subject by an average of 24.6% (range, 4.0-51.2%). Down-regulation of levels of nicotine while smoking in response to infusion of nicotine was imprecise, which may be a result of psychosocial factors influencing smoking behaviour along with the development of tolerance to toxic effects of nicotine as a consequence of prolonged exposure to nicotine. Intravenous nicotine and cigarette smoking increased average heart rate and blood pressure throughout the day and 24-hr urinary epinephrine excretion to a similar extent. Despite higher levels of nicotine when subjects smoked during infusion of nicotine, there were no additional nicotine-related effects.[12]

**<u>David Buck, Antony Morgan</u> (1995)-** A study assessed cessation amongst a representative general adult population in England in order to see whether such aids are as successful amongst more typical smokers. Descriptive information on the pattern of smoking cessation aids use in the English population is presented followed by multivariate analysis of the 'Health in England 1995' survey data set in order to predict successful smoking cessation as a function of several variables including use of nicotine gum and patches, willpower, advice from family physicians, social class, education, gender, marital status and family composition. However, users of nicotine gum and patches were found to be less likely to have given up smoking than non-users. This may be explained by the fact that only those who find it difficult to give up will go to the time and expense of considering such aids because gum and patches were introduced recently in England. Results suggested that 'willpower' is a marker for success in cessation as opposed to a determinant of giving up in its own right. It confirmed a lot of other research on the determinants of smoking cessation and has for the first time looked at the use and impact of nicotine replacement therapy. More research was needed to tease out the true impact of nicotine replacement on cessation rates.[13]

**Analytes to measure tobacco dependence:**

**<u>P. Paoletti* et al</u> (1996)-**A randomized trial was conducted to investigate the effect on outcome of different doses of transdermal nicotine replacement after stratification according to baseline plasma cotinine values. 297 smokers were enrolled. Those with baseline cotinine ≤ 250ngml$^{-1}$ (low cotinine) were randomly assigned to placebo(LC-P) or to 15 mg 16 h nicotine patches (LC-15), and those with baseline cotinine >250 ng·mL$^{-1}$ (high cotinine) were randomly assigned to 15 mg(HC-15) or 25 mg(HC-25) 16 h nicotine patches. Plasma nicotine and cotinine values, expired carbon monoxide and withdrawal symptoms were measured at scheduled intervals during treatment. Smokers in the LC-15 group had a significantly higher success rate than placebo (28 *vs* 9%). Smokers with high baseline cotinine had lower success rates, and a high dose of nicotine did not increase success rate (HC-25 9% *vs* HC-15 11%). Subjects in the HC-15 group had the lowest percentage of nicotine replacement and a higher prevalence of withdrawal symptoms than the HC-25 group. Replacement was similar in groups LC-15 and HC-25, but the success rate was significantly lower in HC-25 group, despite similar levels of withdrawal symptoms. So, a higher success rate was obtained after one year in smokers with low baseline plasma cotinine values. Determination of plasma cotinine values might be helpful in identifying smokers who could benefit from transdermal nicotine replacement.[14]

**Thomas P Moyer et al**- The study was designed to quantify nicotine, cotinine, *trans*-3'-hydroxycotinine, anabasine, and nor nicotine in human serum or urine. The technique required simple extraction of the sample with quantification by HPLC–tandem mass spectrometry. The procedure for simultaneous analysis of nicotine, its metabolites, and tobacco alkaloids simultaneously quantified five different analytes. Test limit of quantification, linearity, imprecision, and accuracy were adequate for clinical evaluation of patients undergoing treatment for tobacco dependency. The test readily distinguished individuals who had no exposure to tobacco products from individuals who were either passively exposed or were abstinent past-tobacco users from those who were actively using a tobacco or nicotine product. Nicotine, cotinine, *trans*-3-hydroxycotinine, nor nicotine, and anabasine could be simultaneously and accurately quantified in either serum or urine by HPLC–tandem mass spectrometry with imprecision <10% at physiologic concentrations and limits of quantification ranging from 0.5 to 5 g/L. Knowledge of serum or urine concentrations of these analytes could be used to guide nicotine replacement therapy or to assess tobacco abstinence in nicotine dependency treatment. These measurements became an integral part of the clinical treatment and management of patients who wish to overcome tobacco dependence.[15]

**Peyton Jacob 3rd et al**-A study was done to determine urine concentration of the tobacco alkaloids anabasine and anatabine, nicotine and its metabolites cotinine, and nor nicotine in 99 cigarette smokers and 205 smokeless tobacco users. They also investigated the possibility that anabasine and anatabine could be used as biomarkers for tobacco use during nicotine replacement therapy. Urine samples and data on self-reported tobacco use were obtained from subjects enrolled in tobacco cessation programs. Urine concentrations of tobacco alkaloids and metabolites were measured and correlated with self reported tobacco use. Concentrations of anabasine and anatabine were used to validate abstinence in smokeless tobacco users who used nicotine gum as part of the therapy. Correlations of alkaloid concentration with self reported tobacco use before treatment ranged from fair to poor. In subjects abstaining from smokeless tobacco but using nicotine gum, anabasine and anatabine levels were below the cut-point of 2ng/ml despite high concentrations of nicotine and cotinine resulting from nicotine gum use. Anabasine and anatabine concentrations in urine could be used to validate abstinence or measure the extent of tobacco use in persons undergoing nicotine replacement therapy.[16]

**R.Croucher et al (2003)-**A short-term longitudinal, quasi-experimental study design was conducted to establish the short-term outcomes for successful tobacco cessation of a programme offering UK resident Bangladeshi women chewing paan with tobacco nicotine replacement therapy (NRT) in addition to brief advice and encouragement alone in the setting of two local authority housing estates in Tower Hamlets, London. Bangladeshi women volunteers were recruited following presentations to community groups. The volunteers were assigned, after matching for age, number of paan with tobacco chewed daily and medical screening, to receive one of two tobacco cessation interventions (NRT with brief encouragement and advice, and brief advice and encouragement alone). The main outcome measures were changes in tobacco use and nicotine dependence, assessed by questionnaire and intake measures, adverse effects, and withdrawal symptoms. In total, 130 volunteers were recruited with mean age 42.5 years (SD =11.3).Mean number of paan quid with tobacco chewed daily was 10.7 (SD =9.3) and the average age of starting to add tobacco to paan was 24 years (SD = 12). Ninety-one percent completed the 4-week trial. They found that 19.5% had stopped tobacco use, of which 22% had received NRT, and 17% brief advice and encouragement alone. The successful members of the NRT group made a significantly greater reduction in their salivary cotinine scores at final review compared to baseline. Methods identified as helping tobacco smokers successfully stop smoking could be used with Bangladeshi women chewing paan with tobacco.[17]

**Craig S. Parzynski et al (2008)**- Cotinine is the most common biomarker used to assess nicotine exposure and abstinence. A study was conducted to examine the relationship between saliva and plasma cotinine concentration in a group of nicotine-dependent adolescent smokers. Additionally, they examined these correlations across gender, ethnicity and age. The sample consisted of 66 adolescent smokers (age 15.1 ± 1.3, 63.6% girls, 66.7% European American, CPD 18.3 ± 8.5, FTND 7.1 ± 1.3). Saliva and plasma specimens were collected before the treatment phase of a nicotine replacement therapytrial and analyzed. The relationship between saliva and plasma cotinine concentration was analyzed using Pearson's correlation coefficients. They performed a secondary analysis using multiple regression. Results indicated a positive correlation between saliva cotinine and plasma cotinine concentration ($r = .84$, $p < .001$). Differences in correlations across age were significant ($t = 3.03$, $p < .01$). Differences across ethnicity approached significance ($t = -1.93$, $p = .058$). Future research should seek to further validate saliva-to-plasma cotinine concentration ratios in adolescents.[18]

**Theresa M Marteau et al (2010)-** An open label, parallel groups randomized trial in which 630 adult smokers (smoking 10 or more cigarettes daily) using National Health Service (NHS), was conducted to estimate the impact upon adherence to nicotine replacement therapy (NRT) of informing smokers that their oral dose of NRT had been tailored to a DNA analysis. Hypotheses to be tested were as follows: I - Adherence to NRT is greater among smokers informed that their oral dose of NRT was tailored to an analysis of DNA (genotype), compared to one tailored to nicotine dependence questionnaire score (phenotype). II- Amongst smokers who fail to quit at six months, motivation to make another quit attempt is lower when informed that their oral dose of NRT was tailored to genotype rather than phenotype. Subjects were randomly allocated to one of two groups: i.) NRT oral dose tailored by DNA analysis (OPRM1 gene) (genotype), or ii.) NRT oral dose tailored by nicotine dependence questionnaire score (phenotype) The primary outcome was proportion of prescribed NRT consumed in thefirst 28 days following an initial quit attempt, with the secondary outcome being motivation to make another quit attempt, amongst smokers not abstinent at six months. Other outcomes include adherence to NRT in the first seven days and biochemically validated smoking abstinence at six months. The primary outcome collected on 630 smokers to detect a 7.5% difference in mean proportion of NRT consumed using a two- tailed test at the 5% level of significance between groups. The proportion of all NRT consumed in the first four weeks of quitting compared between arms using an independent samples t-test and by estimating the 95% confidence interval for observed between-arm difference in mean NRT consumption (Hypothesis I). Motivation to make another quit attempt compared between arms in those failing to quit by six months (Hypothesis II).This was the first clinical trial evaluating the behavioural impact on adherence of prescribing medication using genetic rather than phenotypic information.[19]

**Racial and ethnic variations**

**Steven S. Fu et al (2008)**- A cross-sectional analyses was conducted to examine racial/ethnic variations in the use of nicotine replacement therapy (NRT) and quit ratios among Caucasian, African American, Asian, and Latino lifetime smokers aged 25-44 in individuals (N=27,031) screened for enrollment in the Collaborative Study of the Genetics of Nicotine Dependence (COGEND). Participants were randomly sampled from three Midwestern metropolitan areas from March, 2003 through August, 2005. A telephone survey collected information on smoking history, previous quit attempts, and socio demographic characteristics. Among lifetime smokers (n=9216), univariate analysis indicated that African Americans (22%) and Latinos (22%) were significantly less likely to report having ever used NRT for smoking cessation than Caucasians (31%). Asians (22%) also reported lower rates of using NRT than Caucasians, but this difference was marginally significant ($p$=.06). These disparities persisted in multivariate analysis for African Americans (adjusted OR=0.76, 95% CI=0.63, 0.91, $p<0.01$) but not for Latinos (adjusted OR=0.76, 95% CI=0.54, 1.06, $p$=0.11) or Asians (adjusted OR=0.98, 95% CI=0.60, 1.60, $p$=0.95). As measured by the quit ratio, African Americans (35%) were less likely to have quit smoking than Caucasians (52%). This disparity persisted in multivariate logistic regression (adjusted OR=0.66, 95% CI=0.56, 0.78, $p<0.001$). Asian and Latino smokers were as likely as Caucasians to report smoking cessation. Future prospective studies were needed to assess whether lower utilization of cessation treatments such as NRT contribute to the observed disparity in quit ratios for African Americans. [20]

**William T. Dalton III et al (2010)-**This study was sought to examine patterns of NRT use and risk factors for use to further aid smoking cessation efforts including prevention of potential misuse. In-school surveys assessing socio-demographic and behavioural factors associated with NRT use, gum or patch, were completed by 4078, predominantly African-American, high school students. Approximately 5% of students reported former or current use of NRT products: 42% gum, 29% patch, and 29% both gum and patch. Among smokers, 5.4% reported use of both NRT gum and patch, with exclusive use of gum twice as likely as exclusive use of the patch. Those with high risk-taking attitudes were more likelythan low risk-takers (3% vs. 1%) to report use of both products, with exclusive gum use more prevalent than patch use. A cumulative logit model revealed males, risk takers, and/or smokers were at greatest odds for NRT use.Among this adolescent sample, NRT gum was used more often than the patch. Adolescent males, risk takers, and/or smokers appear more likelyto use NRT (gum and/or patch) compared to their counterparts, despite limited empirical support for effective use of these products as cessation aids among adolescents. Smoking cessation and prevention programs might emphasize appropriate NRT use, specifically within these populations.[21]

**Behavioural Counselling:**

**S.M.Cruse et al (2001)-**GlaxoSmithKline had implemented a voluntary programme of smoking cessation support for its employees in the UK. The 10 week programme offered a series of one-to-one support sessions with a trained occupational health adviser, as well as access to nicotine replacement therapy patches. At 12 months (***n***= 123), 25 participants (20%) were non-smokers, of whom 19 (15%) stated that they had not smoked at all for the 12 month period. The other six (5%) had relapsed, but had since tried again and quit successfully. An additional three (2%) classed themselves as non- smokers but still smoked occasionally. Fifty-two per cent of participants stated that regular face-to-face contact and monitoring of progress were particularly useful in helping them to stop smoking. This provided compelling support for the active promotion and support of smoking cessation among employees.[22]

**David A. Katz et al (2004)-**A randomized, controlled trial of the effectiveness of Guideline implementation at eight community-based primary care clinics in southern Wisconsin (four test & four control sites) was conducted among 2163 consecutively enrolled adult patients who smoked at least one cigarette per day and presented for nonemergency care during the baseline period (June 16, 1999, to June 20, 2000) or the intervention period (from June 21, 2000, to May 3, 2001). The intervention included a tutorial for intake clinicians, group and individual performance feedback for intake clinicians, use of a modified vital signs stamp, an offer of free nicotine replacement therapy, and proactive telephone counselling. Staff at control sites received only general information. Self reported abstinence from smoking was determined by telephone interviews at 2- and 6-month follow-up assessments. Hierarchical logistic regression models were used to estimate the odds ratios (ORs) for treatment assignment after adjustment for patient characteristics. All statistical tests were two-sided. There were no statistically significant differences in smoking cessation rates between participants at test and control sites during the baseline period. Among participants treated during the intervention period, those at test sites were more likely than those at control sites to report being abstinent at the 2-month (16.4% versus 5.8%; adjusted OR = 3.3, 95% confidence interval [CI] =1.9 to 5.6; *P*<.001) and 6-month (15.4% versus 9.8%; adjusted OR = 1.7, 95%CI=1.2to2.6;*P*=.009)follow-up assessments and to report continuous abstinence, i.e. abstinence at both 2 and 6 months (10.9% versus 3.8%; adjusted OR-3.4, 95% CI-1.8 to 6.3; *P*<.001). Implementation of a guideline based smoking cessation intervention by intake clinicians in primary care was associated with higher abstinence among smokers.[23]

**A Molyneux et al (2003)-**A randomised controlled trial of cessation interventions given together compared with counselling alone or minimal intervention was performed in hospital inpatients. Medical and surgical in patients who were current smokers at the time of admission were randomised to receive either usual care (no additional advice at admission), counselling alone (20 minute intervention with written materials), or NRT plus counselling (counselling intervention with a 6 week course of NRT). Continuous and point prevalence abstinence from smoking (validated by exhaled carbon monoxide <10 ppm) was measured at discharge from hospital and at 3 and 12 months, and self-reported reduction in cigarette consumption in smokers was assessed at 3 and 12 months. 274 inpatient smokers were enrolled. Abstinence was higher in the NRT plus counseling group (n=91) than in the counselling alone (n=91) or usual care (n=92) groups. The difference between the groups was significant for validated point prevalence abstinence at discharge (55%, 43%, 37% respectively, p=0.045) and at 12 months (17%, 6%, 8%, p=0.03). There was no significant difference between counselling alone and usual care, or in reduction in cigarette consumption between the treatment groups. NRT given with brief counselling to hospital inpatients was an effective routine smoking cessation intervention.[24]

**Elaine C. Johnstone et al (2007)-** The ATTEMPT cohort was a multinational cohort study with data collection by the internet which recruited smokers of >5 cigarettes per day aged 35–65 years who were intending to stop smoking within the next 3 months. Phase 1 began in spring 2003 and involved 2009 smokers from the USA, UK, Canada and France.

Phase 2 involved 3645 smokers and included the same countries plus Spain. Follow-up assessments were carried out every 3 months. 492 smokers who made a quit attempt without formal behavioural support or bupropion in the first 3-month follow-up period were identified from phase 1, 357 of whom were followed up for a further 6 months. The phase 2 sample involved 906 smokers making quit attempts, 732 of whom were followed up. At baseline, demographic characteristics, smoking history and nicotine dependence were assessed. Smokers who made quit attempts were questioned on methods used to aid them. The main outcome measure was self-report of complete abstinence throughout both the 3-month periods followingthe quit date. 35.6% of smokers followed up in phase 1 and 29.6% of those followed up in phase 2 used NRT. The odds ratios comparing abstinence for 6 months in those using and those not using NRT, adjusting for nicotine dependence, were 3.0 (95% CI 1.2 to 7.5) for the phase 1 sample and 2.1 (95% CI 1.0 to 4.1) for the phase 2 sample. The difference in success rates between those using NRT and those not using it, adjusted for the Fagerstrom test for nicotine dependence (FTND) score, was 6%in the phase 1 sample and 3.7% in the phase 2 sample. NRT use by smokers making self initiated quit attempts without formal behavioural support was associated with improved long-term abstinence rates.[25]

**C. Barr Taylor et al (1996)-**A study was conducted to evaluate a nurse- managed smoking cessation program for smokers hospitalized for a variety of conditions. Hospitalized patients who smoked prior to hospitalization and who were motivated to quit (n=660) were randomized to intervention or usual- care groups and followed for the next year. Intervention included a meeting with nurse care manager; the use of a videotape, workbook, relaxation audiotape, and NRT; and nurse- initiated phone contact after discharge. The 12 month confirmed cessation rates were 21% and 31% for, respectively, the usual- care and intervention group (OR= 1.7; 95% CI= 1.1, 2.3). A nurse- managed smoking cessation intervention can significantly increase cessation rates for hospitalized patients.[26]

**Telephone counselling**

**Robert D. Reid et al (1999)-**A study was conducted at the University of Ottawa Heart Institute to evaluate the incremental efficacy of telephone counselling by a nurse in addition to physician advice and nicotine replacement therapy in helping patients to stop smoking. A total of 396 volunteers who smoked 15 or more cigarettes daily wererandomly assigned to either of 2 groups: usual care (control group) and usual care plus telephone counseling (intervention group); the groups were stratified by sex and degree of nicotine dependence. Usual care involved the receipt of physician advice on 3 occasions, self-help materials and 12 weeks of nicotine replacement therapy. Telephone counselling was provided by a nurse at 2, 6 and 13 weeks after the target quit date. Point-prevalent quit rates were determined at 52 weeks after the target quit date. The point-prevalent quit rates at 52 weeks did not differ significantly between the control and intervention groups (24.1% v. 23.4% respectively). The quit rates did not differ significantly at the secondary measurement points of 4, 12 and 26 weeks. Three additional sessions of telephone counselling by a nurse were ineffective in increasing quit rates. This form of assistance may be useful in the absence of physician advice or when self selected by patients.[27]

**Lawrence C An et al (2006)-**An observational study of cohorts of callers to the Minnesota QUITPLAN$^{SM}$ Helpline before (n = 380) and after (n = 373) the addition of access to free NRT was done to assess change in cessation rates and programme impact after the addition of free nicotine replacement therapy (NRT) to state wide quitline services. The intervention was mailing of NRT (patch or gum) to callers enrolling in multi-session counselling. Thirty-day abstinence six months after programme registration was main outcome measure.The number of callers increased from 155 (SD75) to 679 (180) per month pre-NRT to post-NRT (difference 524, 95% confidence interval (CI) 323 to 725). Post-NRT, the proportion of callers enrolling in multi-session counselling (23.4% v90.1%, difference 66.6%, 95% CI 60.8% to71.6%) and using pharmacotherapy (46.8% v86.8%, difference 40.0%, 95% CI 31.3% to 47.9%) increased.Thirty-day abstinence at six months increased from 10.0% pre-NRT to 18.2% post-NRT (difference 8.2%, 95% CI 3.1% to 13.4%). Post-NRT the average number of new ex-smokers per month among registrants increased from 15.5 to 123.6 (difference 108.1, 95% CI 61.1 to 155.0).The cost per quit pre-NRT was $1362 (SD $207). The cost per quit post-NRT was $1934 ($215) suggesting a possible increase in cost per quit (difference $572, 95% CI 2$12 to $1157).

The addition of free NRT to a state quitline was followed by increases in participation and abstinence rates resulting in an eightfold increase in programme impact. These findings support the addition of access to pharmacological therapy as part of state quitline services.[28]

**Lawrence C An et al (2006)-**New Zealand has a national free-phone Quitline Service which has been operational since 1999. A study was conducted to investigate if the smoke free law increased calls to the Quitline. For 24 months prior to the law, and 12 months after the law, data were collected on: (i) Quitline caller registrations and the issuing of nicotine replacement therapy (NRT) vouchers by the Quitline Service; (ii) expenditure on Quitline-related television advertising; (iii) expenditure on other smoke free television advertising; and (iv) print media coverage of smoking in major New-Zealand newspapers. These data were inputs to a time series analysis using a Box-Jenkins transfer function model. This used the law change as the intervention variable, with the response series being the monthly Quitline caller rates and monthly first time NRT voucher issue rates. The monthly rates of Quitline caller registrations and NRT voucher issues were observed to increase in the months after the law change. The increase in both these outcomes was even greater when considered in terms of per level of Quitline advertising expenditure. In the more robust time series analyses, the law change (intervention variable) had a significant effect ($p = 0.025$) on increasing the monthly caller registration rate in December 2004. This was after adjusting for the possible effects of Quitline advertising expenditure, print media coverage, and other smoking-related advertising expenditure.The new national smoke free law resulted in increased quitting-related behaviour. This would suggest there was an extra opportunity for health agencies to promote quitting at such times.[29]

**Barbara A Schillo et al (2007)-**A study was conducted to describe how the addition of free nicotine replacement therapy (NRT) to the _QUITPLAN Helpline'' in Minnesota influenced triage and transfer to health plan quitlines and how efforts taken to re-establish balance in the partnership expanded population based access to NRT. Call volumes, transfer rates and ClearWay Minnesota dollars spent serving health plan members were examined from May 2001 through November 2005. The process by which health plan quitlines began providing NRT was explored through interviews with health plan representatives. Following the addition of NRT to the QUITPLAN Helpline, the percentage of health plan members transferred to their health plans decreased because callers were resisting transfer to their health plans for telephone counselling that did not include NRT. Transfer rates eventually returned to pre-NRT levels following sequential implementation of scripting changes, transfer requirements and collection of health plan identification numbers. These changes reduced Clear Way Minnesota dollars spent on providing services to insured Minnesotans. Through the partnership, all Minnesotans currently have access to both telephone counselling and NRT either at no or low cost. Minnesota's partnership has effectively expanded access to NRT through quitlines. The increased use of partnerships for providing quitline services might be effective in broadening population access while conserving limited tobacco control dollars for those without cessation benefits.[30]

**David Tinkelman et al (2007)**-A study was conducted to assess the impact on quitline utilisation and cessation outcomes of adding free nicotine patches to the existing programme offerings. Tobacco use status data from the Ohio tobacco quitline were collected from a subset of quitline callers 6 months after the initial intake call. To evaluate the impact of the nicotine replacement therapy (NRT) initiative, quit rates for two groups were compared: those who entered and exited the quitline programme before the availability of free NRT (n = 4657) and those who entered and exited the quitline programme after the availability of free NRT (n = 5715).Call volume increased from 2351 intakes calls per month or 78 calls per day before the availability of free NRT to 3606 intake calls per month or 188 intakes per day following the availability of free NRT ($p<0.0001$). 7-day point prevalence abstinence at 6 months among all quitline callers increased from 10.3% (95% confidence interval (CI) 9.7 to 10.9) before the availability of NRT to 14.9% (95% CI 14.3 to 15.5) after the availability of NRT. Offering free NRT through a state quitline was an effective means of increasing quitline utilization and improving quit rates.[31]

**Jack F Hollis et al (2007)-**A 3x2 randomised trial examined the effectiveness and cost effectiveness of offering callers single session versus multisession counselling, with or without free nicotine patches in 4614 Oregon tobacco quitline callers and compared brief (one 15-minute call), moderate (one 30-minute call and a follow-up call) and intensive (five proactive calls) intervention protocols, with or without offers of free nicotine patches (nicotine replacement therapy, NRT). Blinded staff assessed tobacco use by phone at 12 months. Abstinence odds ratios were significant for moderate (OR = 1.22, CI = 1.01 to 1.48) and intensive (OR = 1.29, CI = 1.07 to 1.56) intervention, and for NRT (OR = 1.58, CI = 1.35 to 1.85). Intent to treat quit rates were as follows: brief no NRT (12%); brief NRT (17%); moderate no NRT (14%); moderate NRT (20%); intensive no NRT (14%); and intensive NRT (21%). Relative to brief no NRT, the added costs for each additional quit was $ 2467 for brief NRT, $ 1912 for moderate no NRT, $2109 for moderate NRT, $264 for intensive no NRT, and $2112 for intensive NRT. Offering free NRT and multisession telephone support within a state tobacco quitline led to higher quit rates, and similar costs per incremental quit, than less intensive protocols.[32]

**C L Miller et al (2009)**-A study was conducted to trial an intervention in a real-life setting to motivate low-income smokers to try to quit. Participants were low-income smokers, recruited "cold" via either a letter in the mail or a flyer inserted in a local newspaper. The intervention group received the usual service of multisession counselling from the quitline plus access to heavily subsidised NRT. A comparison group received the usual quitline service only. Participants were followed up at 3, 6, and 12 months. Trial participants were also compared with a sample of general callers to the quitline. The offer of subsidised NRT recruited more than twice as many low-income smokers than the offer of the cessation service alone (intervention group n=1000; comparison group n=377). 63% were first-time callers to the quitline. Intervention respondents showed higher levels of nicotine dependence than comparison group respondents. 73.5% of smokers in the intervention group tried to quit compared to 61.0% in the comparison group. Unadjusted quit rates were higher in the intervention group than in the comparison group at 3 months and 6 months but not at 12 months. Disadvantaged smokers were easily engaged to call the quitline, particularly when offered subsidized NRT. Disadvantaged smokers using the quitline, with and without subsidized NRT, achieved cessation outcomes comparable to other studies of "mainstream" smokers. [33]

**Jessie E. Saul et al (2011)**-An observational studyevaluated the impact of the Minnesota QUITPLAN® Helpline's shift from distributing NRT using a single eight-week shipment to a two-shipment protocol. Eight week single-shipment cohort (n=247) received eight weeks of NRT (patches or gum) at once, while the split-shipment cohort (n = 160) received five weeks of NRT (n = 94), followed by an additional three weeks of NRT if callers continued with counseling (n = 66). Patient satisfaction, retention, quit rates, and cost associated with the three groups were compared. A higher proportion of those receiving eight weeks of NRT, whether in one or two shipments, reported that the helpline was very helpful than those receiving five weeks of NRT (57.8% of the one-shipment group) ($p = 0.004$). Callers in the eight week two-shipment group completed significantly more calls (3.0) than callers in the five week one-shipment group (2.4) or eight week single-shipment group (1.7) ($p < 0.001$). Using both responder and intent-to-treat calculations, there were no significant differences in 30-day point prevalence abstinence at seven months among the three protocol groups even when controlling for demographic and tobacco use characteristics, and treatment group protocol. The mean cost per caller was greater for the single-shipment phase than the split-shipment phase ($350 *vs.* $326) due to the savings associated with not sending a second shipment to some participants. Assuming no difference in abstinence rates resulting from the protocol change, cost-per-quit was lowest for the five week one-shipment group ($1,155), and lower for the combined split-shipment cohort ($1,242) than for the single-shipment cohort ($1,350). Results indicated that while satisfaction rates increased among those receiving more counseling and NRT, quit rates did not, even when controlling for demographic and tobacco use characteristics. [34]

**Over The Counter availability**

**Saul Shiffman et al (1997)**- A study was conducted to estimate the impact of allowing non- prescription sales of nicotine medications in the United States on increasing the numbers of smoking quitting. Sale and marketing data were used to compare the use of nicotine medications before and after non- prescription sale. Main outcomes measures were number of quit attempts using NRT products, number of smokers who quit smoking with over the counter (OTC) NRT or NRT still sold by prescription, and incremental quits attributable to OTC NRT. Since the Food and drug Administration approved nicotine medications for OTC sale in 1996, use of the medications has increased by 152% compared with prior prescription use. With increased use of an efficacious treatment, OTC nicotine medications are estimated to yield from 11400-30400 new former smokers annually in the United States. The broader availability and promotion of effective treatments for tobacco dependence, specifically gums and patches increase the number of smokers availing themselves of the medications. [35]

**William F Lawrence et al (1998)-**Adecision-analytic model was developed to compare the policy of over-the-counter (OTC) availability of nicotine replacement therapy with that of prescription (Rx) availability for the adult smoking population in the United States. Main outcome measures were long-term (six-month) quit rates, life expectancy, and smoking attributable mortality (SAM) rates. OTC availability of nicotine replacement therapy would result in 91,151 additional successful quitters over a six-month period and a cumulative total of approximately 1.7 million additional quitters over 25 years. All cause SAM would decrease by 348 deaths per year and 2940 deaths per year at six months and five years, respectively. Relative to Rx nicotine replacement therapy availability, OTC availability would result in an average gain in life expectancy across the entire adult smoking population of 0.196 years per smoker. In sensitivity analyses, the benefits of OTC availability were evident across a wide range of changes in baseline parameters. Compared with Rx availability of nicotine replacement therapy, OTC availability would result in more successful quitters, fewer smoking-attributable deaths, and increased life expectancy for current smokers. [36]

**Mark B. Reed et al (2005)-**A study used data from the 1996 California Tobacco Survey to compare the rates of nicotine replacement therapy (NRT) use and smoking abstinence in California for each month during a period immediately preceding and immediately following the OTC availability of nicotine gum and patches. For smokers eligible to report a quit attempt, the proportion making a quit attempt using NRT and the proportion remaining abstinent was calculated for each of the 12 months prior to the survey interview. Multiple regressions modelling of quit attempts and abstinence included a term for the number of months between the quit attempt and survey interview and dummy variables for the months before and after the OTC availability of NRT. Results showed a significant increase in the fraction of smokers using the patch ($P < 0.01$) and gum ($P < 0.05$) immediately following their availability OTC. There was also a significantly higher proportion of smokers reporting abstinence with gum use ($P < 0.01$) and a significant increase in reported abstinence with patch use ($P<0.01$) during the period of time immediately following the availability of these products without a prescription. It suggested that removing the prescription status of NRT products resulted in an immediate increase in quit attempts and smoking abstinence with the use of nicotine gum or patches. [37]

**R West et al (2005)-**A study used sales data to examine the impact of government initiatives to increase access to smoking cessation medicines. Information about prescription and non-prescription sales (1999–2002) was obtained. Estimates of utilisation were compared with findings from the Office of National Statistics (ONS) omnibus surveys. The effects of policy initiatives (making the medicines reimbursable and making them available on general sale outside pharmacies) were assessed by means of time series analysis. In addition a new nicotine replacement therapy (NRT) product (a nicotine lozenge) was launched and the effect of this on total utilisation was assessed. Making bupropion, and subsequently nicotine replacement therapy (NRT), reimbursable had a major impact in medication usage; the estimated increase in each case was more than 80 000 "treatment weeks" purchased per month. In addition, introduction of a nicotine lozenge increased total utilisation and did not detract from usage of other medicines. According to both the sales and the survey data, the proportion of smokers using medicines to aid smoking cessation more than doubled from 8–9% in 1999 to 17% in 2002. The ONS surveys showed no increase in the proportions of smokers making quit attempts and so the effects were solely on the proportions of quit attempts that were aided by medication. In the UK, making smoking cessation medicines reimbursable led to alarge increase in utilisation. While the effect on smoking prevalence would be too small to be detected in national surveys it could have a substantial public health impact. [38]

**Kristina B.Metzger et al (2005)-**NewYork City and NewYork State increased cigarette excise taxes and New York City implemented a smoke-free workplace law. To assess the impact of these policies on smoking cessation in New York City, a study examined over-the-counter sales of nicotine replacement therapy (NRT) products. Pharmacy sales data were collected in real time as part of non-traditional surveillance activities. They used Poisson generalized estimating equations to analyze the effect of smoking-related policies on pharmacy-specific weekly sales of nicotine patches and gum. They assessed effect modification by pharmacy location. They observed increases in NRT product sales during the weeks of the cigarette tax increases and the smoke-free workplace law. Pharmacies in low income areas generally had larger and more persistent increase in response to tax increase than those in higher-income areas. Real-time monitoring of existing non traditional surveillance data, such as pharmacy sales of NRT products, could help assess the effects of public policies on cessation attempts. Cigarette tax increase and smoke-free workplace regulations were associated with increased smoking cessation attempts in New York City, particularly in low-income areas. [39]

**Kristina B. Metzger et al (2002)-**A study was conducted to examine trends in smoking cessation, pharmaceutical cessation aid use, and success in cessation in the general California population.The large population-based California Tobacco Surveys of 1992, 1996, and 1999, including 5247 (71.3% response rate), 9725 (72.9% response rate), and 6412(68.4% response rate) respondents, respectively. Main outcome measures were Rates of cessation attempts (>1 day) among smokers in the last year, use of pharmaceutical aids (mostly over-the-counter products since 1996), and cessation success. Between 1992 and 1999, cessation attempts among California smokers increased 61.4% (from 38.1% to 61.5%), and NRT use among quitters increased 50.5% (from 9.3% to 14.0%). A total of 17.2% of quitters used NRT, an antidepressant, or both as an aid to cessation in 1999. In 1996 and 1999, the median duration of aid use (14 days) was much less than recommended, and only about 20% of users had adjuvant one-on-one or group behavioural counselling. Use of NRT increased short-term cessation success in moderate to heavy smokers in each survey year. A long term cessation advantage was only observed before NRT became widely available over the- counter (August 1996). Since becoming available over the counter, NRT appeared no longer effective in increasing long-term successful cessation in California smokers. [40]

**S Shiffman et al (2003)-**A study was conducted to estimate the incidence of persistent use of over-the-counter( OTC) nicotine gum and patch for periods of > 3 months, > 6 months, > 12 months, and > 24 months in a national panel of 40 000 US households, 2690 recorded NRT purchases. Analysis of NRT purchase patterns in data from a population based panel of US households that electronically scanned all household purchases between January 1997 and March 2000. Among 805 households that purchased nicotine gum, 2.3% of new purchase incidents led to continuous monthly purchase of gum for >6 months. For

Nicotine patches (2050 households), the percentage was 0.9%.For both gum and patch, the incidence of persistent purchase dropped below 0.4% by 24 months. Allowing one month gaps within a "continuous" purchase run resulted in increased estimates (for gum: 6.7% for>6 months and 1.0% for>24 months; for patch: 1.7% for>6 months and 0.05% for> 24 months).Persistent use of nicotine gum and patch was very rare and had not increased with the transition to OTC use, despite removal of physician oversight. [41]

**Anne N. Thorndike et al (2002)-**A study was conducted to examine whether the change in nicotine replacement therapy sales from prescription to over the counter (OTC) status affected smoking cessation. Study used the 1993–1999 Massachusetts Tobacco Surveys to compare data from adult current smokers and recent quitters before and after the OTC switch. No significant change over time occurred in the proportion of smokers who used nicotine replacement therapy at a quit attempt in the past year (20.1% pre-OTC vs 21.4% post-OTC), made a quit attempt in the past year (48.1% vs 45.2%), or quit smoking in the past year (8.1% vs 11.1%). Fewer non-Whites used nicotine replacement therapy after the switch (20.7% pre-OTC vs 3.2% post-OTC, $P = .002$), but the proportion of Whites using nicotine replacement therapy did not change significantly (20.6% vs 24.0%).It observed no increase in Massachusetts smokers' rates of using nicotine replacement therapy, making a quit attempt, or stopping smoking after nicotine replacement therapy became available for OTC sale. There appear to be other barriers to the use of nicotine replacement therapy besides visiting a physician, especially among minority smokers. [42]

**Anne N. Thorndike et al (2003) -**Cross-sectional survey of 4078 high school students during the school term of 1998 in City schools in Memphis, Tenn was done to report the prevalence, ease of access and reasons for NRT use and describe inappropriate use in adolescent smokers and non smokers. Main Outcome Measures were Community-based self reported prevalence of NRT use and characteristics of those using NRT. Approximately 5% of adolescents reported trying or using nicotine gum or patches. Females were less likely than males and African Americans were less likely than others to use NRT. For African American smokers, NRT use was highest at lower smoking levels, while other smokers showed the opposite pattern. Almost 40% of former smokers reported using NRT to try to quit smoking; however, 75% of current smokers endorsed using NRT for reasons other than trying to quit smoking. Other inappropriate use of NRT was reported; 18% of NRT users reported themselves as never smokers. More than 50% of students reported that it would be easy for them to get NRT. Nicotine replacement therapy was used by adolescent smokers and non smokers, was easily accessible, and was used for reasons other than trying to quit smoking. Efforts are needed to discourage NRT use in non smoking youth and to encourage appropriate use of NRT in young smokers to maximize its potential for successful cessation.[43]

**The-wei Hu et al (2000)-** Astudy was conducted to examine the effect of sales of nicotine replacement products on national cigarette consumption. National time series quarterly cigarette consumption, sales of nicotine gums and patches data between 1976 and 1998 were used to estimate a time series autoregressive moving average intervention model. Main outcome measures were Per capita cigarette sales.A 10% increase in sales of nicotine replacement products will lead to a 0.04% reduction in cigarette sales. The model indicates that a 0.076% reduction in cigarette consumption was associated with the availability of nicotine patches after 1992. Nicotine replacement products (nicotine gums and nicotine patches) play a significant role in reducing cigarette consumption, in addition to the negative effect of increasing cigarette price and the overall trend of declining cigarette consumption (as reflected by the time trend variable). This study suggested that additional efforts for promoting sales of nicotine replacement products will be another effective alternative to discouraging cigarette consumption. [44]

**Effectiveness of NRT**

**Karl Olov Fagerstrom et al (1997)-**A study was conducted in 143 men and women smoking an average of 22.6(SD 7.0) cigarettes per day and exhibiting a Fagerstrom Tolerance Questionnaire score of 7.0 ( SD 1.9), to assess the effect of the various nicotine replacement therapy ( NRT) on smoking reduction. During an initial sampling week subjects familiarized with nicotine gum, patch, nasal spray, vaporizer and sublingual tablet. A cross over design was used during the next 4 study weeks. They were randomly assigned a product to use. Subjects were asked to use as much NRT as they wished, yet to smoke enough to feel comfortable. Main outcome measure were Self-reported cigarette consumption, exhaled carbon monoxide (CO), withdrawal symptom score, cotinine plasma levels and motivation to quit were monitored over a period of five weeks. Self- reported smoking declined steadily over the five weeks, from 22.6 (SD7.0) to 10.4 (SD

1.0) ($P<0.001$) cigarettes daily (54% decrease). Smoking reduction was greater on average during the weeks when the subjects could choose their nicotine product than when products were assigned. CO readings decreased confirming a reduction in smoking (35% decrease), although cotinine levels remained steady, suggesting that subjects were titrating nicotine to their original levels. Withdrawal scores decreased over time (32% decrease, $P<0.001$), showing that there was no discomfort associated with the smoking reduction, and motivation to quit was enhanced by the treatment in most subjects (93%). NRT for aiding smoking reduction appeared to be safe, was associated with a clinically significant reduction in smoke exposure over a five-week follow up, and increased motivation to stop smoking.[45]

**S Shiffman et al (2005)-**Mail survey of US smokers from a national research panel to assess differences in demographic and smoking characteristics between smokers who had and had not used nicotine replacement therapy (NRT) in smokers 18 years and over who returned a survey on smoking (n = 9630). The sample was weighted to match the US smoker population on age and sex. They compared quit attempt on demographic characteristics, nicotine dependence, history of craving and withdrawal, expected difficulty quitting, and self reported history of smoking related medical illness and psychopathology. NRT users (both ever-users and OTC users) were more likely to be older, male, and better educated. They were also heavier smokers, had experienced more craving and withdrawal upon quitting, and scored higher on measures of dependence. These differences were evident among light smokers, and remained even when smoking rate and time to first cigarette were controlled. Smokers who elect to use NRT differ from non-NRT users in ways that predispose them to failure in cessation. Controlling for smoking rate and time to first cigarette does not eliminate these differences, even among light smokers. These differences must be considered when comparing the effectiveness of NRT among samples of smokers who self selected their treatment and were likely to bias such outcome comparisons. [46]

**John A. Cunningham et al (2008)-**A study was conducted to determine intentions of smokers to use free nicotine replacement therapy. A telephone survey of 825 randomly selected daily smokers aged 18 years or older who had smoked at least 10 cigarettes per day at some point in their lives.Overall, 58.9% of the respondents said they would be interested in nicotine replacement therapy if it were offered for free. Of those interested, almost all (93.8%) said that they would use the nicotine replacement therapy to help them quit for good. There were differences in the levels of interest: smokers who intended to quit were more interested in using the nicotine replacement therapy than those who planned to reduce or maintain their smoking. [47]

**John A Cunningham et al (2011)-**A single blinded, panel survey design with random assignment to an experimental and a control condition was conducted to determine wide public health initiatives NRT distribution in Canada and other countries through the mail. A two-stage recruitment process employed, in the context of a general population survey with two follow-ups (8 weeks and 6 months). Random digit dialing of Canadian home telephone numbers identified households with adult smokers who were willing to take part in a smoking study that involved three interviews, with saliva collection for 3-HC/cotinine ratio measurement at baseline and saliva cotinine verification at 8-week and 6-month follow-ups (N=3,000).Eligible subjects interested in free NRT determined at baseline (N = 1,000) and subsequently randomized into experimental and control conditions to receive versus not receive nicotine patches. The primary hypothesis was that subjects who receive nicotine patches will display significantly higher quit rates at 6-month follow-up as compared to subjects who do not receive nicotine patches at baseline. The findings from the proposed trial were timely and highly relevant as mailed distributions of NRT require considerable resources and there were limited public health dollars available to combat this substantial health concern. In addition, it informed the development of models to engage smokers to quit, incorporating proactive recruitment and the offer of evidence based treatment. [48]

**Nancy Amodei & R. J. Lamb (2010)-** An exploratory study examined whether voluntary early use of NRT predicted cessation in a self-initiated quit attempt better than other commonly studied variables. Data were collected from 99 adult smokers desiring to quit smoking in the near future over a 10-day baseline period prior to the implementation of a contingency management intervention. NRT use was neither encouraged nor discouraged during the study. Initial abstinence, biochemically verified using a criterion of CO level<4 ppm, was conceptualized in 2 ways: (a) any day of baseline abstinence and (b) the sum of baseline days abstinent. They examined the predictive value of NRT use as well as demographics, self-efficacy, motivational readiness, and nicotine dependence. While greater self-efficacy was predictive of initial abstinence, NRT use was the most consistent predictor. The odds of abstaining at least 1 day during baseline were 16.8 times greater for those who used NRT on Day 1 than nonusers. Self –efficacy and "any baseline NRT use" contributed significant amounts of variance to the "sum of days abstinent," with the overall model explaining 29% of the variance ($p < .001$). The sum of baseline days of NRT use and use of NRT on Day 1 also predicted the "sum of days abstinent." Given NRT's effectiveness, but under utilization in real-world settings, the data support the need for interventions or strategies encouraging people to use NRT in their quit attempts. [49]

**Chris Bullen et al (2006)-**Prospective pragmatic uncontrolled clinic-based pilot study was done to test the acceptability and tolerability of using NRT while smoking for two weeks before quitting in 14 adult smokers recruited from a smoking cessation clinic were prescribed nicotine patches or gum with follow up for two weeks. Data were collected on participants'concerns about smoking while using NRT, importance of quitting, urges to smoke, smoking behaviour, previous NRT use and the length of the pre-quitting period. Urine tests were collected weekly for cotinine, and participants recorded smoking activity and noted experiences and changes in their health in diaries. Only 21% of 14 participants expressed concerns about using NRT while smoking. All of the nine followed up used it as recommended, 56% of these reporting no unpleasant symptoms. Median urine cotinine levels declined over the two weeks. Urges to smoke averaged 1.8 on a 4 point scale. All participants decreased the number of cigarettes per day. Diary records showed wide variation in smoking and NRT use,with an increased sense of control and determination to quit.Smokers using pre-quitting NRT over two weeks appeared to titrate nicotine levels and symptoms of toxicity were uncommon and of low intensity. [50]

**Effect of NRT on Profile of Mood States (POMS):**

**Tellervo Korhonen et al (2006)-**A study evaluated the effects of Nicotine Replacement Therapy (NRT) on the Profile of Mood States (POMS), testing whether pre-cessation depressive symptoms modify NRT's effects on POMS. Out of 608 smokers attempting to quit with NRT, this secondary analysis included 242 participants abstinent for at least two weeks. They measured pre-cessation depressive symptoms with the Centre for

Epidemiological Studies Depression Scale. At 1, 7, and 14 post-cessation days, they examined 6 self-reported POMS, i.e.feeling 'anxious', 'sad', 'confused', 'angry', 'energetic' and 'fatigue'. The results of the ANCOVA models suggested no NRT effects on feeling anxious, energetic or fatigue. They found that pre-cessation depression modified NRT effects in some specific mood states, such as depression by NRT-interaction effects on feeling confused and feeling angry. On average, the depressed participants in the placebo groups had the highest symptom scores. However, those depressed in NRT conditions did not have significantly higher symptom scores compared to the non-depressed groups. In treating those negative moods NRT might be particularly important for persons with depressive symptoms before cessation.[51]

**NRT and systemic conditions**

**Douglas M. Ziedonis and Tony P. Qeorge (1997)**-Nicotine's action and the pathobiology of schizophrenic disorders have common neurobiological substrates. Tobacco smoking alters medication blood levels and effectiveness, modifies psychiatric symptoms, and is a clue for other substance abuse. This study presented an evaluation of a smoking cessation program for 24 smokers with schizophrenia. Fifty percent completed the program, 40 percent decreased use by 50 percent, and 13 percent remained abstinent (carbon monoxide verified) for 6 months. Nicotine replacement, motivational enhancement therapy, and relapse prevention behavioural therapy were important components of treatment. Pharmacotherapy strategies of a higher-dose nicotine patch, combining nicotine gum and a patch, and augmentation medication to nicotine replacement should be evaluated in future studies in this population. [52]

**R Hubbard et al (2005)**-Self control case series analysis of data from The Health Improvement Network (THIN) (a computerized general practice database) estimated the relative incidence of myocardial infarction and stroke in four 14 day periods before and after the first prescription for NRT in Patients contributing data to THIN. This observational study of NRT measured Acute myocardial infarction, acute stroke, and death. 33 247 individuals had been prescribed NRT, of whom 861 had had a myocardial infarction and 506 a stroke. There was a progressive increase in the incidence of first myocardial infarction in the 56 days leading up to the first NRT prescription (overall incidence ratio 5.55, 95% confidence interval (CI) 4.42 to 6.98), but the incidence fell after this time and was not increased in the 56 days after starting NRT (incidence ratio 1.27, 95% CI 0.82 to 1.97). The results were similar for second myocardial infarction and stroke, and for subgroups of people with pre-existing angina and hypertension.There were 960 deaths in this cohort during a mean follow up period of 2.6 years after starting NRT, with no evidence of an increased mortality in the 56 days after the NRT prescription (incidence ratio 0.86, 95% CI 0.60 to 1.23).The use of NRT was not associated with any increase in the risk of myocardial infarction, stroke, or death. [53]

**Michael D. Stein et al (2006)-**A study was conducted to determine the association between daily smoking and use of nicotine replacement therapy (NRT), and to determine predictors of greater NRT use among 383 methadone-maintained smokers at five methadone maintenance treatment centres. Intervention was to assign free nicotine patch (8 to 12 weeks) plus either a baseline-tailored brief motivational intervention, a quit date behavioural skills counselling session, and a relapse prevention follow- up session (max), or brief advice using NCI's 4 A's model (min). 309 (80.6%) set a specific quit date (received NRT) and were located for assessments. Participants were 51.8% male, 78.6% Caucasian, and smoked 26.6 (SD=12.2) cigarettes/day. On the day following their quit day, 86.4% of participants used NRT. The percentage of participants using NRT was 52.3%, 27.1%, and 10.4% on day 30, day 60, and day 90 respectively. Participants used NRT on 44.1% of the days through the 90 days of the treatment protocol. The estimated odds of smoking abstinence was 7.1 (P<.001) times higher on days when NRT was used than on days when NRT was not used, and cigarettes/day was also significantly lower on NRT days (14.93 vs 4.65; P<.001). Nicotine replacement therapy use was inconsistent following an initial quit attempt among methadone-maintained smokers. On days when NRT was used, individuals were likely to smoke at reduced levels or not at all.[54]

**Tim Coleman et al (2004)-**A study was conducted to determine i) the feasibility of recruiting women to a RCT of NRT in pregnancy as they attend hospital antenatal ultrasound examinations, ii) the proportion of such women who are eligible for and interested in trial enrolment and iii) research staff perceptions of how one method of trial recruitment could be improved. During a one month period, all women attending for antenatal ultrasound examination in an English teaching hospital were asked to complete a questionnaire which determined their eligibility to enroll in a proposed placebo controlled randomized trial investigating the effectiveness of NRT in pregnancy. Over 99% (851/858) of women agreed to complete a questionnaire about smoking habits. 10.3% (88/851) of women attending for antenatal ultrasound fitted eligibility criteria for a proposed RCT of NRT in pregnancy, but only 3.6% [(31/851), 95% CI, 2.4 to 4.9%] indicated on the questionnaire that they would like to take part in a study involving randomization to placebo or active patches. Researchers offered trial enrolment to 26 of these 31 women and 96% (25) accepted. Staff recruiting women believed that trial recruitment would be maximized if women attending the ultrasound department knew about trial recruitment before attending and greater staff resources were made available for this. It was also perceived that women generally under-reported the amount they smoked on questionnaires completed whilst waiting in ultrasound department areas. It was feasible to recruit women for a trial of NRT in pregnancy as they wait for antenatal ultrasound examinations. [55]

**Ioanna Milidou et al (2012)-**A study was conducted to investigate the associations between use of nicotine replacement therapy (NRT) and smoking during pregnancy and infantile colic in the offspring. They used data from maternal interviews (from pregnancy and at 6 months post partum) from the Danish National Birth Cohort (1996–2002). They included 63,128 live-born single tons with complete information on nicotine exposure during pregnancy and infantile colic symptoms as recorded at 6 months of age. A total of 46,660 infants (73.9%) were unexposed to nicotine during pregnancy; 207 (0.3%) were exposed to NRT, 15,016 (23.8%) were exposed to smoking, and 1245 (2.0%) to both. A total of 4974 (7.9%) infants fulfilled Wessel's modified criteria for infantile colic. Prenatal nicotine exposure was associated with elevated risk for infantile colic in the offspring. Compared with the unexposed, NRT users had an adjusted odds ratio (OR) (95% confidence interval) of 1.6 (1.0– 2.5; P = .03), smokers had OR = 1.3 (1.2–1.4), and women who both smoked and used NRT had OR = 1.6 (1.3–1.9). They corroborated the association between smoking and infantile colic after adjustment for several possible confounders in a large cohort study. Moreover, they found that infants exposed to NRT prenatally had an increased risk for infantile colic of the same magnitude as those exposed to tobacco smoke. Thus, nicotine might play a role in the pathogenesis of infantile colic. [56]

**Tim Coleman et al (2012)-**A study was conducted to investigate the efficacy and safety of nicotine patches during pregnancy. They recruited participants from seven hospitals in England who were 16 to 50 years of age with pregnancies of 12 to 24 weeks' gestation and who smoked five or more cigarettes per day. 1050 participants received behavioral cessation support and were randomly assigned to 8 weeks of treatment with active nicotine patches (15 mg per 16 hours) to 521 or matched placebo patches to 529 participants. The primary outcome was abstinence from the date of smoking cessation until delivery, as validated by measurement of exhaled carbon monoxide or salivary cotinine. Safety was assessed by monitoring for adverse pregnancy and birth outcomes. There was no significant difference in the rate of abstinence from the quit date until delivery between the nicotine-replacement and placebo groups (9.4% and 7.6%, respectively; unadjusted odds ratio with NRT, 1.26; 95% confidence interval, 0.82 to 1.96), although the rate was higher at 1 month in the nicotine-replacement group than in the placebo group (21.3% vs.11.7%). Compliance was low; only 7.2% of women assigned to nicotine-replacement therapy and 2.8% assigned to placebo used patches for more than 1 month. Rates of adverse pregnancy and birth outcomes were similar in the two groups. Adding a nicotine patch (15mg per 16 hours) to behavioral cessation support for women who smoked during pregnancy did not significantly increase the rate of abstinence from smoking until delivery or the risk of adverse pregnancy or birth outcomes. However, low compliance rates substantially limited the assessment of safety.[57]

**Public Health Aspects**

**Martin Lindstrom (2007)-**A cross-sectional survey was done in 2004 public health in Skane, Sweden in which a total of 27,757 people aged 18–80 answered a postal questionnaire. The participation rate was 59%. Different strategies to support smoking cessation—that is, no therapy, nicotine replacement (NRT), professional therapy and snus (snuff) use, were investigated among quitters according to year of smoking cessation, and demographic and socioeconomic characteristics. 14.9% of the men and 18.1% of the women were daily smokers. The prevalence of daily snus use was 19.5% among men but only 2.3% among women. Stratifying the data according to year of smoking cessation (1938–2004) revealed a significant increase in active smoking cessation strategies such as NRT, professional therapy and snus use. NRT was more common among women (23.6%) than men (14.8%) among smokers who quit in 2000–4, but snus use was more common among men (30.4% versus 8.7%). No replacement or other therapy at all was significantly more common among women (63.6%) than men (52.1%). People aged 35–80 years used more nicotine replacement than people aged 18–34, while men aged 18–34 used snus to quit smoking significantly more than men aged 55–80. Snus was used commonly among men as a support for smoking cessation in Sweden. Women used pharmacological NRT to a greater extent, but this could probably not compensate for the much higher extent of snuff use as a cessation strategy among men. [58]

**Anne N. Thorndike et al (1998)-**A study was done by 3254 physicians recorded data on 1,45,716 adult patient visits to assess recent trends in the treatment of smokers by US physicians in ambulatory care and to determine whether physicians'practices meet current standards. Design was based on analysis of 1991-1995 data from the National Ambulatory Medical Care Survey, an annual survey of a random sample of US office-based physicians. Main outcome measures were the proportion of visits at which physicians (1) identified a patient's smoking status, (2) counselled a smoker to quit, and (3) used nicotine replacement therapy. Smoking counselling by physicians increased from 16% of smokers' visits in 1991 to 29% in 1993 (P<.001) and then decreased to21% of smokers' visits in 1995 (P<.001). Nicotine replacement therapy use followed a similar pattern, increasing from 0.4% of smokers' visits in 1991 to 2.2% in 1993 (P<.001) and decreasing to 1.3% of smokers' visits in 1995 (P=.007). Proportion of physicians identified patients' smoking status at 67% of all visits in 1991, did not increase over time. All physicians were more likely to treat patients with smoking-related diagnoses. Although a transient peak in counselling and nicotine replacement use occurred in 1993 after the introduction of the nicotine patch. In particular, patient visits for diagnoses not related to smoking represented important missed opportunities for intervention.[59]

**A Wilson etal (2005)-**A prospective cohort study using practices registered with the pilot QRESEARCH database was done to compare the characteristics of smokers who do and do not receive smoking cessation treatment in primary care in 1,56,550 patients aged 18 years and over from 39 general practices located within four strategic health authorities in UK. Subjects were patients who registered with practices between 1 April 2001 and 31 March 2003 aged 18 years and over who were identified as smokers before the two year study period.Of the 29, 492 patients recorded as current smokers at the start of the study period 1892 (6.4%) were given prescriptions for smoking cessation treatment during the subsequent two years. Of these, 1378 (72.8%) were given NRT alone, 406 (21.5%) bupropion alone, and 108 (5.7%) both treatments. Smokers were more likely to receive smoking cessation treatment if they lived in the most deprived areas (odds ratio (OR) for the most relative to the least deprived fifth, adjusted for sex, age, and co-morbidity, 1.50, 95% confidence interval (CI) 1.26 to 1.78), and if they were aged 25–74 years comparedto 18–24 years or 75 and over. Smokers with co-morbidity were also more likely to receive smoking cessation treatment. Smokers were less likely to receive smoking cessation treatment if they were male (adjusted OR 0.68, 95% CI 0.62 to 0.75). The low proportion of smokers being prescribed these products strongly suggested that a major public health opportunity to prevent smoking related illness was being missed.[60]

**Michael K. Ong et al (2005)-**A study was conducted to compare the cost- effectiveness of a free nicotine replacement therapy (NRT) program with a statewide smoke-free workplace policy in Minnesota. They conducted 1-year simulations of costs and benefits. The number of individuals who quit smoking and the quality-adjusted life years (QALYs) were the measures of benefits. After 1 year, a NRT program generated 18,500 quitters at a cost of $ 7020 per quitter ($4440 per QALY), and a smoke-free workplace policy generated 10400 quitters at a cost of $799 per quitter ($506 per QALY).Smoke-free workplace policies are about 9 times more cost-effective per new nonsmoker than free NRT programs are.Smoke-free workplace policies should be a public health funding priority, even when the primary goal is to promote individual smoking cessation.[61]

**Benjamin J.Apelberg et al (2010)-**A study was conducted to compare potential population-wide benefits and risks.They examined the potential impact of increased nicotine replacement therapy (NRT) use for smoking cessation on future US mortality. They developed a simulation model incorporating aMonte Carlo uncertainty analysis, with data from the 2005 National Health Interview Survey and Cancer Prevention Study II. It estimated the number of avoided premature deaths from smoking attributable to increased NRT use, before and after incorporating assumptions about NRT harm. Result showed gradual increase in the proportion of NRT-aided quit attempts to 100% by 2025 would lead to 40000 (95% credible interval= 31000, 50000) premature deaths avoided over a 20-year period. Most avoided deaths would be attributable to lung cancer and cardiovascular disease. After they incorporated assumptions about potential risk from long-term NRT, the estimate of avoided premature deaths from all causes declined to 32000. Even after assuming some harm from long-term NRT use, the benefits from increased cessation success far outweigh the risks. However, the projected reduction in premature mortality still reflected a small portion of the tobacco-related deaths expected over a 20-year period. [62]

**Jonathan P. Winickoff et al (2003)-**A study was conducted to evaluate the feasibility of implementing a smoking cessation intervention for parents at the time of the paediatric visit. A prospective cohort of smoking parents whose child was seen in an outpatient paediatric practice was offered the Stop Tobacco Outreach Program, which includes 3 brief counselling sessions, written materials, free nicotine replacement therapy (NRT), proactive referral to a Free State telephone quit line, and fax referral to the parents' primary clinician. The primary outcome was completion of all three counselling sessions. Other outcomes were quit attempts, cessation, NRT use, state quit line use, and household smoking assessed at 2-month follow-up. 158 smoking parents met eligibility criteria and 100 (63%) enrolled in the study. Of the 100 enrolles, 81% completed all three counselling sessions and 78% accepted free NRT at the time of enrollment. At 2-month follow-up, of the 100 enrolles, 56% reported making a quit attempt of >24 hours, 18% reported 7-day tobacco abstinence, 34% used NRT, and 42% received additional counselling from the state telephone quit line. The mean number of cigarettes smoked inside the home and car declined over 2 months. This study demonstrates the feasibility of engaging parents in a smoking cessation intervention at the time of a child's clinic visit. This approach might be an effective way to reach smokers who otherwise are unlikely to access smoking cessation interventions.[63]

**Elin Roddy et al (2006)-**A study was conducted to determine whether nicotine replacement therapy (NRT) when combined with counselling was effective in young smokers in a deprived area of Nottingham, UK. They surveyed smoking prevalence and attitudes to smoking and quitting in young people accessing an open access youth project in a deprived area of Nottingham, and used the information gained to design a community based smoking cessation service incorporating a randomized controlled trial of nicotine patches against placebo given in association with individual behavioural support. They resurveyed smoking prevalence among project attendees after completing the pilot study.

Of 264 young people surveyed (median age 14 years), 49% were regular smokers. A total of 98 young people were recruited and randomized to receive either active nicotine patches on a six week reducing dose regimen, or placebo. Adherence to therapy was low, the median duration being one week, and 63 participants did not attend any follow up. At four weeks, five subjects receiving active NRT and two receiving placebo were abstinent, and at 13 weeks none were. Adverse effects were more common in the active group but none were serious. Smoking prevalence among 246 youth project attendees surveyed after the trial was 44%.It suggested that NRT in this context was unlikely to be effective in young smokers and also suggested that young smokers wanted help with smoking cessation, but establishing the efficacy of smoking cessation services for young people who need them most, would be very difficult.[64]

**Tobacco Cessation Centres**

**Abu Saleh M. Abdullah et al (2004)-**A study was done to evaluate a pilot smoking cessation health centre (SCHC) of the Hong Kong Council on Smoking and Health (COSH).Smokers were recruited mainly by low cost publicity. Trained counsellors provided individual counselling and a 1 week free supply of nicotine replacement therapy (NRT). The programme was evaluated in terms of process, outcome and cost. During August 2000 to January 2002, 2212 calls were received through the clinic hotline and1203 smokers attended the clinic. Eight hundred and forty-one were successfully followed up at 12 months. Based on intention-to treat analysis, the 7 day point prevalence quit rate at 12 months (not smoking any cigarette during the past 7 days at the 12 month follow-up) was 27 percent (95 percent, CI25–30 percent). The average cost per quitter was US $339 (US $440 including NRT cost for a 1week free supply).Other benefits included training of healthcare workers and medical students, organization of seminars, health talks and promotion of research and training. This first evaluation of a clinic-based smoking cessation service in Asia showed that the service was acceptable to Chinese smokers. The quit rate in this pilot part-time clinic was comparable to those of full-time and better funded clinics in the West. A part-time smoking cessation clinic was a promising model for piloting smoking cessation services in the East. [65]

**Cherian Varghese et al(2012)-**In the beginning 2002, a network of 19 tobacco cessation clinics (TCCs) was set up over a period of time to study the feasibility of establishing tobacco cessation services. Review of the process and operational aspects of setting up TCCs was carried out by evaluation of the records of TCCs in India. Baseline and follow-up information was recorded on a pre-designed form. During a five-year period, 34,741 subjects attended the TCCs. Baseline information was recorded in 23 320 cases. All of them received simple tips for quitting tobacco; 68.9% received behavioural counseling for relapse prevention and 31% were prescribed adjunct medication. At six-week follow-up, 3255 (14%) of the tobacco users had quit and 5187 (22%) had reduced tobacco use by more than 50%. Among 12 813 patients, 26% had either quit or significantly reduced tobacco use at first follow-up (three-months), 21% at the second (six-months) and 18% at the third follow-up (nine-months) had done so. This study concluded that it is feasible to set up effective tobacco cessation clinics in developing countries. [66]

## VARIOUS NICOTINE REPLACEMENT THERAPY AGENTS:

### SILVER ACETATE:

**R Malcolm et al (1986)-**A double-blind controlled study was conducted using Silver acetate chewing gum, a non prescription medication which produces an unpleasant metallic taste in the mouth of individuals who consume tobacco products in conjunction with this smoking deterrent. Its use leads to self-induced aversive conditioning. Subjects using silver acetate for three weeks of treatment had a smoking cessation rate of 15 out of 136 (11 %, p=0.02) whereas placebo subjects had a smoking cessation rate of 6 out of 146 (4 %, p = .102) Without further treatment, silver acetate group demonstrated a 7% non smoking rate at four months compared with 3 % non smoking rate for the placebo group. Silver acetate demonstrated a modest benefit over placebo as a smoking deterrent in a minimal intervention and highly cost-effective treatment setting.[67]

**E J Jensen et al (1990)-**A randomized study of comparison of the effect of silver acetate, nicotine, and ordinary chewing gum on smoking cessation was conducted on 196 smokers. All were motivated to stop smoking abruptly and all had smoked at least 10 cigarettes a day for at least five years. The participants attended nine meetings over a year, at which lectures, support, and advice about stopping smoking were given. Tobacco abstinence was confirmed by measurement of carbon monoxide in expired air. After 12 weeks there was a trend towards more abstainers in the nicotine group (59%) than in the silver acetate (50%) and ordinary (45%) chewing gum groups that was not quite significant (p = 0 07). At 26 and 52 weeks the number of cigarette abstainers was similar in the three treatment groups. Subjects in the nicotine chewing gum group had a longer mean time before relapse than those in the silver acetate and ordinary chewing gum groups. Mean success rates for all subjects combined at 12, 26, and 52 weeks were 52.8%, 39.7%, and 23.3%. The side effects of nicotine and silver acetate chewing gum were mild and transient except for mouth irritation from silver acetate and the low taste acceptability of nicotine, which had a strong negative influence on the success rate. The results suggested a short term effect of nicotine chewing gum on smoking cessation, but the abstinence rates after one year were generally disappointing. [68]

**NICOTINE GUM:**

A physician's prescription used to be required to obtain the gum, but in 1996 the gum became an over-the-counter (OTC) medication. Nicorette is the brand name but there are generic forms of the gum. The manufacturer states that Nicorette allows smokers to self-titrate (up to 24 pieces a day) and it is currently available in six different flavours. The gum allows the nicotine to be absorbed through the mucus membranes of the mouth between the cheek and the gums. It comes in a 4 milligram (mg) dose for those patients who smoke more than 25 cigarettes a day and a 2 mg dose for those who smoke less than 25 cigarettes a day.

**Directions** One piece of nicotine gum is chewed every one to two hours at first, or it may be chewed when you have the urge to smoke. Chew slowly until you can taste the nicotine or feel a slight tingling in your mouth.Then stop chewing and place the gum between your cheek and gum. When the tingling sensation is almost gone (about 1 minute), start chewing again. Repeat this procedure for about 30 minutes. Do not chew more than one piece of gum at a time. Gradually reduce the amount of nicotine gum after two to three months. Reducing the use of nicotine gum over time will help prevent withdrawal symptoms.

**Tips to help reduce the use of nicotine gum gradually include**

- Decrease the total number of pieces used per day by about one piece every four to seven days.
- Decrease the chewing time with each piece from the normal 30 minutes to 10 to15 minutes for 4 to 7 days. Then gradually decrease the total number of pieces per day.
- Substitute pieces of nicotine gum with one or more pieces of sugarless gum for an equal number. Every four to seven days, increase the number of sugarless gum pieces as substitutes for nicotine gum.
- Replace the 4-mg gum with the 2-mg gum and apply the previous steps.
- Consider stopping use of nicotine gum when your craving for nicotine is satisfied by one or two pieces of gum per day.

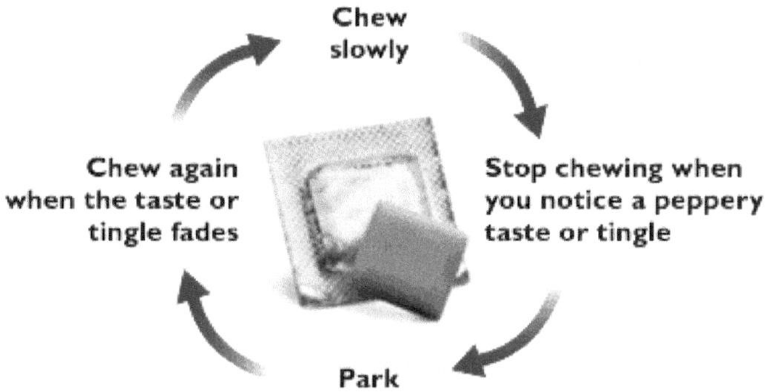
Chew
slowly
Stop chewing when
you notice a peppery
taste or tingle
Park
Chew again
when the taste or
tingle fades

**M J Jarvis et al (1982)-**A double-blind randomized trial was conducted to check the effectiveness of 2 mg nicotine chewing-gum as an aid to stop smoking as compared to a placebo containing 1mg nicotine, but un buffered. Of 58 subjects given the active gum, 27 (47%) were not smoking at one-year follow-up compared with 12 (21%) of the 58 subjects treated with placebo ($p<0.025$). 18 (31%) subjects in the active treatment group and eight (14%) in the placebo group had not smoked at all from the start of treatment to follow-up at one year ($p <005$). Subjects receiving the active gum experienced less severe withdrawal symptoms and rated their gum as more helpful than did the placebo group. Minor side effects were common but only gastric symptoms were more frequent with the active gum. Subjects receiving active gum used it for longer than those receiving placebo but most stopped using it within six months and only four (7%) developed longer-term dependence. The number of gums used daily correlated significantly with pre treatment blood nicotine concentrations in the active treatment group and with pre treatment cigarette consumption in the placebo group. A lower pre treatment blood nicotine value was the best predictor of success at one year ($p <0\ 001$) but there was no significant relation to cigarette consumption, sex, and social class. The results confirmed the usefulness of nicotine chewing-gum as an aid to stop smoking and imply a definite role for nicotine in cigarette dependence and withdrawal. [69]

**M A H Russell et al (1983)-**A study was designed to see whether the offer and prescription of nicotine chewing gum would enhance the efficacy of general practitioners' advice to stop smoking. A sample of 1938 cigarette smokers who attended the surgeries of 34 general practitioners in six group practices were assigned by week of attendance to one of three groups: (a) non intervention controls, (b) advice plus booklet, and (c) advice plus booklet plus the offer of nicotine gum. Follow up was done after four months and one year. The results showed a clear advantage for those offered the nicotine gum (p <0001). The proportions who were abstinent at four months and still abstinent at one year were 39%, 41%, and 88% in the three groups, respectively. The effect of the offer and prescription of gum was to motivate more smokers to try to stop, to increase the success rate among those who tried, and to reduce the relapse rate of those who stopped. The self selected subgroup of 8% who used more than one box of 105 pieces of gum achieved a success rate of 24%. It would be feasible and effective for general practitioners to include the offer of nicotine gum and brief instructions on its use as part of a minimal intervention routine with all cigarette smokers.Such a routine could expect to achieve about 35-40 long term ex-smokers a year and so save the lives of about 10 of them. If replicated by all general practitioners throughout the country, the yield of ex-smokers would be about one million a year. [70]

**Konrad Jamrozik et al (1984)-**A study was conducted on 2110 adult cigarette smokers to see the effect of antismoking advice in general practice, 429 who reported at follow up after one year that they had tried unsuccessfully to stop smoking were offered "a special antismoking chewing gum,"either nicotine gum or a placebo gum, in a double blind study. Of 200 who were willing to try the gum, 101 were randomly allocated to the nicotine gum and 99 to the placebo gum. They were followed up at six months by an unannounced home visit, at which they were interviewed and asked to provide a breath sample for analysis of carbon monoxide. Twenty five claimed that they had stopped smoking, but, of them, seven exhaled levels of carbon monoxide indicative of continued smoking. Of the 18 in whom giving up smoking was validated, 10 had received active gum and eight placebo gum, a difference which was not significant (odds in favour of nicotine gum = 1.25, 95% confidence limits 0.47-3.31). The value of nicotine chewing gum, if any, can be quite small when it is used in general practice.[71]

**A I Hjalmarson (1984)-**The effect of 2-mg nicotine chewing gum as an adjunct to group therapy for smoking cessation was studied in a placebo-controlled, double-blind, randomized trial. After one year, 29% of the 106 subjects treated with nicotine chewing gum had remained abstinent throughout the year compared with 16% of the

99 subjects treated with placebo. The results were confirmed by measurement of levels of expired CO. More subjects in the nicotine group (70/94 *v* 45/93) reported that the gum reduced the craving for smoking. The adverse effects were few and not serious. In the nicotine group, 3% were still using the nicotine gum after two years. No subjects in the placebo group used the chewing gum beyond six months. Nicotine chewing gum is effective in improving the success rates in smoking cessation based on group therapy.[72]

**Richard Leigh et al (2001)-** A 12-week, prospective, double-blind, randomized, placebo controlled pilot study to determine whether combination of sublingual pralidoxime and ipratropium ProBAN together with nicotine replacement improves quit rates compared with nicotine replacement alone at University-affiliated outpatient clinic. Of 107 subjects seen at the screening visit, 27 were excluded because of comorbid illness or concomitant medication use. Of 80 eligible subjects, 40 were randomly assigned to receive treatment with ProBAN sub- lingual tablets and nicotine gum (treatment group), and 40 to receive placebo tablets and nicotine gum (control group) for 12 weeks. The primary outcome was complete continuous abstinence of smoking from one through 12 weeks after the quit date. There were no adverse effects in the treatment group. At one week after the quit date, 35% of ProBAN-treated subjects had quit compared with 18% of control subjects (odds ratio [OR] 2.5, 95% CI 0.9 to7.2).Corresponding quit rates at four weeks were 28% and 15% (OR 2.1, 95% CI 0.7 to 6.5), at eight weeks were 25% and 13% (OR 2.3, 95% CI 0.7 to 7.6), and at 12 weeks were 23% and 13% (OR 2.0, 95% CI 0.6 to 6.7), respectively. ProBAN combined with nicotine replacement doubled the continuous sustained quit rate compared with nicotine replacement alone, with no adverse effects. Although not statistically significant due to the size of the study, this result suggests that it may be an effective therapy for smoking cessation, and larger studies are warranted. [73]

**Anna B Jessen et al (2003)-**A randomized, double-blind, placebo-controlled, crossover study included 12 healthy, normal-weight men (aged 18–45 y) was done to assess the acute thermogenic effects of chewing gum containing different doses of nicotine and caffeine. Energy expenditure was measured with indirect calorimetry before and 2.5 h after subjects chewed each of 7 different types of gum containing the following doses of nicotine/caffeine: 0/0, 1/0, 2/0, 1/50, 2/50, 1/100, and 2/100 mg/mg. The thermogenic responses (increases over the response to placebo) were 3.7%, 4.9%, 7.9%, 6.3%, 8.5%, and 9.8%, respectively, for the gums containing 1/0, 2/0, 1/50, 2/50, 1/100, and 2/100 mg nicotine/mg caffeine ($P < 0.05$ for all). Adding caffeine to 1 and 2 mg nicotine significantly enhanced the thermogenic response, but changing the caffeine dose (from 50 to 100 mg) did not change the thermogenic effect. None of the combinations changed the respiratory quotient compared with placebo, which indicated that glucose and fat oxidation rates were increased to a similar extent. One milligram of nicotine had a pronounced thermogenic effect, which can be increased by~100% by adding 100 mg caffeine. Increasing the nicotine dose to 2 mg did not increase the thermogenic effect but produces side effects in most subjects. Caffeine might be useful in preventing weight gain after smoking cessation if its thermogenic effect can be used to enhance nicotine's effect on long-term energy balance.[74]

**Mayumi Mochizuki et al (2004)-**A randomized, controlled study was done to evaluate whether pharmacists' advice on smoking cessation would result in a higher smoking cessation rate using Nicorette (nicotine gum preparation). Fourteen pharmacies in Japan participated. Smokers who visited pharmacies to buy Nicorette from March 1, 2002, through August 31, 2002, were recruited and randomly assigned to two groups. For the intervention group (A) (n=11), pharmacists provided both regular instructions on Nicorette use and smoking cessation advice at the first sale and then gave follow-up advice just before starting a cessation and 1, 3, and 8 weeks and 3 months thereafter. For the control group (B) (n=17), pharmacists provided regular instructions alone. The primary outcome measure was the self-reported smoking cessation rate and the secondary outcome measure was the relationship between the smoker's egogram and effectiveness of intervention. The absolute abstinence rate in groups A and B at 3 months was 45.5% and 31.2%, respectively. The odds ratio was 1.83, which was not statistically significant. There was no difference in ego gram score between absolute abstinence subjects and non abstinence subjects in group A. The egogram scores in Adapted Child of absolute abstinence subjects in group B were significantly higher than in non abstinence subjects. In conclusion, instructions and advice given by pharmacists might improve the smoking cessation rate in smokers receiving nicotine replacement therapy.[75]

**Cheryl Oncken et al (2008)-**To estimate the safety and efficacy of treatment with 2 mg nicotine gum for smoking cessation in pregnant women who smoked daily received individualized behavioural counseling and random assignment to a 6-week treatment with 2 mg nicotine gum or placebo, followed by a 6-week taper period. Women who did not quit smoking were instructed to reduce the number of cigarettes smoked by substituting with gum. Measures of tobacco exposure were obtained throughout the study. Participants in the nicotine (N=100) and placebo (N=94) groups were comparable in age, race/ethnicity, and smoking history.Biochemically-validated smoking cessation rates were not significantly higher with nicotine replacement therapy compared with placebo (after 6 weeks of treatment: 13% vs.9.6%, p=.45; at 32-34 weeks of gestation: 18% vs 14.9%, p= .56). Using a completer analysis, nicotine replacement therapy significantly reduced the number of cigarettes per day [nicotine replacement therapy: -5.7 (SD=6.0); placebo: -3.5 (SD=5.7); p=.035], and cotinine concentration [nicotine replacement therapy: -249 ng/mL (SD=397); placebo: -112 ng/mL (SD=333); p=.04]. Birth weights were significantly greater with nicotine replacement therapy vs. placebo [3287 g (SD=566 and 2950 g (SD=653, respectively; p<.0001]. Gestational age was also greater with NRT than placebo (38.9 wk [SD=1.7] and 38.0 wk [SD=3.3], respectively; p=.014). Despite not reducing smoking during pregnancy, use of nicotine gum increased birth weight and gestational age, two key parameters in predicting neonatal wellbeing.[76]

## TRANSDERMAL NICOTINE PATCHES

The patch comes in four main brands: Nicotrol, Nicoderm, Prostep, and Habitrol. All four patches transmit low doses of nicotine to the body throughout the day. Other smoking cessation programs or materials should be used while using the patch. One patch contains 21mg of nicotine and is recommended for patients who smoke more than 10 cigarettes per day. Another patch contains 14 mg of nicotine and is recommended for patients who smoke less than 10 cigarettes per day.

### Directions

Apply the patch directly to the skin once a day, usually at the same time of day. Apply the patch to a clean, dry, hairless area of skin on the upper chest, upper arm, or hip, as specified by the package directions. Remove the patch from the package, peel off the protected strip, and immediately apply the patch to your skin. Press the patch to the skinby placing the palm of your hand over it for about 10 seconds. Be sure the patch is held firmly in place, especially around the edges. Wash your hands with water only after applying the patch. Wear the patch continuously for 16 to 24 hours. Remove the patch carefully, and dispose off it by folding it in half with the sticky sides touching. After removing the patch, apply the next patch to a different skin area to prevent skin irritation. Nicotine patches maybe used from 6 to 20 weeks. A switch to a lower strength patch may be considered after the first two weeks. A gradual reduction to a lower dosage of the patch is recommended so that the amount of nicotine in the system is reduced and consequently, the nicotine withdrawal symptoms will be reduced.

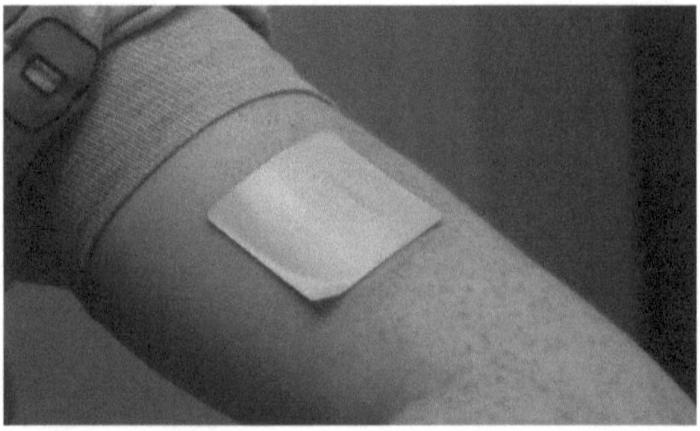

A two 6-week, randomized, double-blind, placebo-controlled, parallel group trials were conducted to evaluate the efficacy of a new transdermal nicotine system for smoking cessation in nine specialized outpatient clinics. Successful abstainers from both trials enrolled in a third trial for blinded down titration from medications (6 weeks) and subsequent off-drug follow-up (12 weeks). Subjects were healthy volunteers who smoked one or more packs of cigarettes daily and wanted to participate in a smoking cessation program. Patients were randomly assigned to a transdermal nicotine system delivering nicotine at rates of 21, 14, or 7 mg (in trial 1 only) over 24 hours or to placebo. Group counselling sessions were provided to all participants. Rates of continuous smoking abstinence were determined during 6 weeks of full-dose treatment, a 6-week weaning period (through week 12), and a 3-month follow-up receiving no therapy (through week 24). Abstinence was defined by patient diary reports of no smoking during the designated periods, confirmed by expired-breath carbon monoxide levels of 8 ppm or lower. Cessation rates during the last 4 weeks of the two 6-week trials were 61%, 48%, and 27% for 21-and 14-mg transdermal nicotine and placebo, respectively ($P \leq .001$ for each active treatment vs placebo). Six-month abstinence rates for 21-mg transdermal nicotine and placebo were 26% and 12%, respectively ($P \leq .001$). All transdermal nicotine doses significantly decreased the severity of nicotine withdrawal symptoms and significantly reduced cigarette use by patients who did not stop smoking.Compliance was excellent, and no serious systemic adverse effects were reported. Transdermal nicotine systems showed considerable promise as an aid to smoking cessation.[77]

**D M Daughton et al (1991)-**A double-blind, placebo-controlled trial was conducted in 158 smokers to assess the smoking cessation efficacy of transdermal nicotine patches as an adjunct to low-intervention therapy. Participants were randomly assigned to one of the following three study regimens that required daily application of two $15 cm^2$ patches: (1) 24-hour nicotine delivery, (2) nicotine delivery during wakeful hours only, and (3) placebo. The impact of the three regimens on smoking cessation rates and tobacco withdrawal symptoms was examined.During the last 2 weeks of the trial, 39% of the 24-hour nicotine regimen delivery group, 35% of those on wakeful hour nicotine regimens, and 13.5% of the placebo treatment group achieved abstinence. Self-reported quit rates for the two nicotine patch-wearing regimens, as compared with that for the placebo group, continued to be significantly higher at 6 months. Compared with placebo, the transdermal nicotine patches significantly reduced tobacco withdrawal symptoms during the first few weeks of quitting.The differences in quit rates and tobacco withdrawal symptoms between the two active groups were not statistically significant.The patches were well tolerated both topically and systemically.So, transdermal nicotine, when used as an adjunct to low-intervention therapy, significantly reduced tobacco withdrawal symptoms and enhanced smoking cessation rates.[78]

**MA H Russell et al (1993)-**A randomised double blind placebo controlled parallel group study with one year of follow up was done to evaluate the efficacy of transdermal nicotine patches as an aid to stop smoking when used as an adjunct to brief advice and support in a general practice setting in 30 general practices in 15 English counties. Subjects were 600 dependent heavy smokers (> 15 cigarettes daily) who were well motivated to give up. Brief general practitioner advice, booklet, and 16 hours per day patch treatment for 18 weeks with brief support and follow up at one, three, six, 12, 26, and 52 weeks. Self reported complete abstinence for up to one year with biochemical validation at all follow up points. Nicotine patches reduced the severity of craving and adverse mood changes in the first weeks of withdrawal and doubled the rate of initial cessation at week 3 (nicotine group 36% of patients, placebo group 16.5% of patients) and of continuous abstinence throughout one year (nicotine group 9.3%, placebo group 5.0 %). A dose increase at week 1 among patients experiencing difficulty in quitting increased the proportion who achieved abstinence at week 3. There were no adverse systemic effects attributable to nicotine, but the incidence of moderate or severe local irritation or itching at the patch site was 16.4% (63 patients), compared with 3.8% (7) with placebo. Transdermal nicotine patches used as an adjunct to brief advice and support in a general practice setting are an effective aid to long term cessation of smoking in highly dependent smokers.[79]

**PL Yudkin et al (1996)-**A randomized, double-blind, placebo controlled trial of nicotine transdermal patches were analysed retrospectively to examine whether the effectiveness of transdermal patches is related to nicotine dependence or to other smoker characteristics and to investigate factors predicting smoking cessation using patches in 1686 patients recruited from 19 general practices in Oxfordshire. The main outcome was continuous smoking cessation from 8 to 52 weeks after the start of patch use, biochemically validated at 12, 24 and 52 weeks. Nicotine transdermal patches were more effective in smokers with moderate nicotine dependence [odds ratio (OR) 1.94; 95% confidence interval (Cl) 1.24 - 3.04] than in mildly or highly dependent smokers (OR 0.98; 95% Cl 0.58-1.65) and more effective in those aged 24-49 years (OR 1.89; 95% Cl 1.24 - 2.87) than in older smokers aged 50-65 years (OR 0.88; 95% Cl 0.49 - 1.59). Abstinence from smoking in the first week of the trial was the strongest predictor of sustained cessation and was more common among smokers using nicotine patches than those using placebo patches (33% of 842 compared with 22% of 844; P<0.001).Of first week abstainers, 25 and 28% of 277 and 182 in the nicotine and placebo groups, respectively, achieved sustained cessation compared with 4% of 565 and 2% of 662 first-week smokers. Nicotine transdermal patches were most effective for smokers with moderate nicotine dependence and for younger smokers. A week's trial of the patch proceeding to longer term use if abstinence was achieved might be an effective policy.[80]

Lowell C. Dale et al (1995)-A Randomized, double-blind clinical trial was done to examine weight change in subjects receiving variable doses of transdermal nicotine replacement for smoking cessation in One-week inpatient treatment with outpatient follow-up through 1 year. Weight change was examined after smoking cessation for 70 subjects randomized to placebo or to 11, 22, or 44mg/d doses of transdermal nicotine.The study included 1 week of intensive inpatient treatment for nicotine dependence with active patch therapy continuing for another 7 weeks. Counselling sessions were provided weekly for the 8 weeks of patch therapy and with long-term follow-up visits at 3, 6, 9, and 12 months. Forty-two subjects were confirmed biochemically (i.e., by expired carbon monoxide) to be nonsmokers at all weekly visits during patch therapy. Their 8 week weight change from baseline was 3.0 +/- 2.0 kg. For these subjects, 8-week weight change was found to be negatively correlated with percentage of cotinine replacement (r=-.38,p = .012) and positively correlated with baseline weight(r = .48, p = .001), and age (r = .35, p=.025). Men had higher (p=.003) 8-week weight gain (4.0+/-1.8kg) than women (2.1 +/-1.7kg).Of the 21 subjects who abstained continuously for the entire year, 20 had their weight measured at 1-year follow-up. This study suggested that higher replacement levels of nicotine may delay post cessation weight gain for both men and women. It could not identify any factors that predict weight change with long-term abstinence from smoking.[81]

**John P Shaw et al (1998)-**A study was conducted to assess nicotine patch use in smokers who purchased the product as a non-prescription medicine from pharmacies. A questionnaire was administered at the time of purchase at Community pharmacies throughout New Zealand to 805 male and female purchasers of nicotine patches aged 18 through 87 years. Main outcome measures were patterns of usage including self-reported smoking history, previous quit-smoking attempts, previous and current use of transdermal nicotine and other products, side effects, and concomitant smoking. Most respondents (74%) had attempted to quit smoking previously, many of whom (53%) had used a non-prescription nicotine replacement product. Approximately 60% of purchasers were first-time users. Twenty-eight per cent of respondents reported continuing smoking while using transdermal nicotine, although thenumber of cigarettes smoked was much less, than in the reported smoking history. Side effects were reported by 24% of patch users in the current course, but there was no evidence of significant safety problems. This survey provides preliminary data on the non-prescription usage of transdermal nicotine when purchased through pharmacies.[82]

**N L Benowitz et al (1998)-**A study was conducted to test the hypothesis that transdermal nicotine, dosed up to three times the doses currently recommended for smoking cessation, would suppress nicotine intake from *ad libitum* smoking in a dose-dependent manner. Eleven volunteers with no desire to quit smoking received placebo or 21, 42, and 63 mg/day transdermal nicotine, with and without cigarette smoking, in a blinded crossover study. Cigarette smoking was permitted as desired. Transdermal nicotine suppressed nicotine intake from cigarette smoking by 3%, 10% and 40% on average in the 21, 42 and 63 mg/day conditions. The number of cigarettes smoked per day declined from an average of 17.2 to 12.7 and the intake of nicotine per cigarette declined from 2.5 to 1.6 mg, comparing placebo and 63 mg nicotine conditions. Results suggested that high-dose transdermal nicotine has the potential to substantially suppress the intake of tobacco smoke and could be a useful strategy for smoking cessation therapy or for reducing the harm caused by smoking.[83]

**Ubirani Barros Otero et al (2006)-**Randomized clinical trial carried out to investigate the effectiveness of the cognitive-behavioural approach and nicotine replacement therapy with nicotine patches for smoking cessation. Participated 1,199 adults, volunteers, in Rio de Janeiro, Brazil, randomly assigned to 10 different groups: intensive brief counselling group (GB), with 1 or 2 sessions (G1-G2), and with 3 or 4 sessions (G3-G4), with/without nicotine replacement therapy (NRT). Abstinence proportions were estimated during 12 months. These proportions among participants not assigned to NRT were 20% (GB), 17% (G1-G2), and 23% (G3- G4); and among assigned NRT groups were 30% (GBA), 34% (G1A-G2A), and 33% (G3A-G4A). After multiple adjustments, the abstinence proportions ratios seemed to follow a "dose-response" pattern: compared to GB, the ratios were 0.85 (G1-G2), 1.13(G3-G4), 1.51(GBA), 1.66(G1A-G2A), and 1.75(G3A-G4A). The results suggested that use of NRT increases the abstinence proportion for cessation. The "dose-response" pattern suggested that cognitive-behavioural could be the reasonable option in the smoking cessation therapy.[84]

**Dorothy Hatsukam et al (2007)-**Adose-ranging,within subject design was implemented to evaluate the effects of 15, 30 and 45 mg nicotine patch treatment on measures of safety and the extent of smoking reduction and biomarker exposure per cigarette in smokers (*N* = 20 completers) not immediately interested in quitting. Concurrent smoking and NRT were generally tolerated and resulted in no changes in blood pressure or heart rate. Slightly less than 10% of the study sample was not given the highest dose of NRT due to side effects. Self-reported cigarette smoking decreased with increasing doses of nicotine replacement and significant reductions were observed for total NNAL (a carcinogen biomarker) and carbon monoxide. However, even at the 45 mg dose, increased carbon monoxide and total NNAL per cigarette occurred, even though cotinine levels increased on average, 69.3% from baseline. The results suggested that the use of high dose NRT is safe, leads to significant reductions in smoking (-49%), significant but less reductions in total NNAL (-24%) and carbon monoxide (-37%) due to compensatory smoking.[85]

**Jon O. Ebbert et al (2007)-**A randomized, placebo-controlled clinical trial was conducted to obtain preliminary evidence on the safety and efficacy of high dose nicotine patch therapy among smokeless tobacco (ST) users who consume ≥ 3 cans of ST per week with 42 ST users randomized to nicotine patch doses of 21, 42, and 63 mg/day or placebo. Serum nicotine concentrations were measured during *ad libitum* ST use and nicotine replacement therapy, and percentages of nicotine replacement were calculated. They observed substantial inter-subject variability in nicotine concentrations with *ad lib* ST use.

The mean percentage replacement of *ad lib* ST use serum nicotine concentrations approximated 100% with the 42mg/day patch dose (mean ± SD, 98.4% ± 45%). Dosing with the 21 mg/day nicotine patch was associated with mean "under-replacement" (53.2%±17.1%), and the 63 mg/day nicotine was associated with mean "over-replacement" (159.2% ± 121.9%). They observed symptoms of nausea consistent with nicotine toxicity in two subjects in the 63 mg/d group while no subjects in the 42 mg/d reported toxicity symptoms. The use of 42 mg/day nicotine patch therapy is safe and should be considered as initial therapy in the clinical setting among ST users who use ≥ 3 cans per week.[86]

**SP David et al (2008)-**Smokers of European ancestry (*n* = 720) who participated in a double-blind, randomised, placebo controlled trial of transdermal nicotine replacement therapy, were genotyped for two functional polymorphisms (variable number of tandem repeats (VNTR) and a C to T transition at position −521 (C-521T)) in the dopamine D4 receptor gene (*DRD4*) gene. Logistic regression models of abstinence at 12- and 26-week follow-ups were carried out separately for each polymorphism. For the *DRD4* VNTR models, the main effect of treatment was significant at both 12-week ($P = 0.001$) and 26-week ($P = 0.006$) follow-ups, indicating an increased likelihood of successful cessation on active nicotine replacement therapy transdermal patch relative to placebo. The main effect of *DRD4* VNTR genotype was associated with abstinence at 12-week follow-up ($P = 0.034$), with possession of one or more copies of the long allele associated with reduced likelihood of cessation (17 vs 23%), but this effect was not observed at 26-week follow-up. For the *DRD4* C-521T models, no main effect or interaction terms involving genotype were retained in themodels at either 12-or 26-week followup. These data were consistent with observations from studies of the *DRD2* gene that genetic variants related to relatively decreased dopaminergic tone in the mesocorticolimbic system were associated with increased risk for relapse to smoking following a cessation attempt.[87]

**Irene M. Glenn and Jesse Dallery et al (2007)-**An experiment compared the short-term effects of a transdermal nicotine patch to voucher-based reinforcement of smoking abstinence on cigarette smoking. Fourteen heavy smokers (7 men and 7 women) completed the four 5-day phases of the study: baseline, patch treatment, voucher treatment, and return to baseline. The order of the two treatment phases was counter balanced across participants. In the patch treatment condition, participants wore 14-mg transdermal nicotine patch every day. In the voucher treatment condition, participants received vouchers contingent on abstinence from smoking, defined as producing carbon monoxide (CO) readings of #4 parts per million. Participants e-mailed two video clips per day showing them breathing into a CO monitor and the resulting CO reading to clinic staff. In the voucher treatment, 24% of samples were negative, and 5% of samples were negative in the patch treatment. Results suggested that contingent vouchers were more effective than transdermal nicotine patches in promoting abstinence.[88]

**Elaine C. Johnstone et al (2007)-**A double-blind, randomized, placebo-controlled trial of the nicotine transdermal patch between June 1991 and March 1992 was conducted in 1,686 patients from general practice (GP) surgeries in Oxfordshire, United Kingdom to determine the association of *catechol* O-*methyltransferase* (*COMT*) genotype with abstinence following a smoking cessation attempt among a large cohort of smokers who attempted to quit using either the nicotine transdermal patch or placebo and were followed up over an 8-year period following their initial cessation attempt. In addition, they examined the possible moderating influence of sex on any association. The genotype × treatment interaction effect at 12-week follow-up indicated a greater benefit of active nicotine replacement treatment compared with placebo on likelihood of abstinence in the *COMT* Met/Met genotype group (33% versus 12%), in comparison to the Met/Val + Val/Val group (22% versus 16%). Results indicated that *COMT* genotype might moderate the effect of active transdermal nicotine patch compared with placebo, with reduced relative benefit of nicotine replacement therapy in individuals with Met/Val or Val/Val genotype. It suggested that genetic variation in the dopamine pathway might provide a future basis for tailored smoking cessation therapies, but indicated that different genes influencing various components of this pathway might have different effects on response to smoking cessation pharmacotherapy.[89]

**Rana Abu-Huwaij et al (2011)-**An in-vitro study was conducted to observe the feasibility of formulating mucoadhesive buccal patches that demonstrate a fast initial release and a lateral, prolonged controlled release that satisfy the needs for smoking cessation. Bilayer nicotine mucoadhesive patches were prepared and evaluated to determine the feasibility of the formulation as a nicotine replacement product to aid in smoking cessation. Nicotine patches were prepared using xanthan gum or carbopol 934 as a mucoadhesive polymers and ethyl cellulose as a backing layer. The physicochemical interactions between nicotine and the polymers were investigated by Fourier transform infrared (FTIR) spectroscopy. Mucoadhesion was assessed using two-arm balance method, and the in vitro release was studied using the Franz cell. FTIR revealed that there was an acid base interaction between nicotine and carbopol as well as nicotine and xanthan. Interestingly, the mucoadhesion and in vitro release studies indicated that this interaction was strong between the drug and carbopol whereas it was weak between the drug and xanthan. Loading nicotine concentration to non-medicated patches showed a significant decrease in the mucoadhesion strength of carbopol patches and no significant effect on the mucoadhesion strength of xanthan patches. In vitro release studies of the xanthan patches showed a reasonable fast initial release profile followed by controlled drug release over a 10-h period.[90]

**GUMS AND PATCHES:**

**Jin Ling Tang et al (1994)-**A study was conducted to assess the efficacy of nicotine replacement therapy in helping people to stop smoking. Analysis of the results of 28 randomised trials of nicotine 2 mg chewing gum, six trials of nicotine 4 mg chewing gum, and six trials of nicotine transdermal patch was done. Nicotine 2 mg chewing gum had an overall efficacy of 6% (95% confidence interval 4% to 8%), greater in self referred subjects than in invited subjects (11% v 3%). Efficacy depended on the extent of dependence on nicotine as assessed by a simple questionnaire; it was 16% (7% to 25%) in "high dependence" smokers, but in "low dependence" smokers there was no significant effect. The 4 mg gum was effective in about one third of "high dependence" smokers. The efficacy of the nicotine patch (9% (6% to 13%) overall) was less strongly related to nicotine dependence, perhaps because the patch cannot deliver a bolus of nicotine to satisfy craving. Both gum and patch are effective aids to help nicotine dependent smokers who seek help in stopping. Among the most highly nicotine dependent smokers the 4 mg gum was the most effective form of replacement therapy; it could enable one third to stop. In less highly dependent smokers the different preparations are comparable in their efficacy but the patch offers greater convenience and minimal need for instruction in its use. Overall, nicotine replacement therapy could enable about 15% of smokers who seek help in stopping smoking to give up the habit.[91]

**Ned L. Cooney et al (2009)-** A study was conducted to compare the efficacy of smoking cessation treatment using the combination of active nicotine patch plus active nicotine gum versus therapy consisting of active nicotine patch plus placebo gum in a sample of alcohol dependent tobacco smokers in an early phase of outpatient alcohol treatment and also to determine whether or not there were any carry over effects of combination nicotine replacement on drinking outcomes. Small scale randomized double-blind placebo controlled clinical trial with one-year smoking and drinking outcome assessment at two outpatient substance abuse clinics provided a treatment platform of behavioural alcohol and smoking treatment delivered in three months of weekly sessions followed by three monthly booster sessions in 96 men and women with a diagnosis of alcohol abuse or dependence and smoking 15 or more cigarettes per day. All participants received open-label transdermal nicotine patch and were randomized to receive either 2 mg nicotine gum or placebo gum under double blind conditions. Analysis of 1-year follow-up data revealed that patients receiving nicotine patch plus active gum had better smoking outcomes than those receiving patch plus placebo gum on measures of time to smoking relapse and prolonged abstinence at 12 months. Alcohol outcomes were not significantly different across medication conditions. Results of this study were consistent with results of larger trials of smokers without alcohol problems showing that combination therapy (nicotine patch plus gum) was more effective than monotherapy (nicotine patch) for smoking cessation.[92]

### 3.4.D NASAL NICOTINE INHALAR

The inhaler should be used with a smoking cessation program, which may include support groups, counselling, or specific cognitive and behavioural therapies. Nicotine oral inhalation comes as a cartridge to inhale by mouth using a special inhaler.

**Directions**

Your doctor may increase or decrease your dose depending on your urge to smoke. The inhaler has a plastic mouthpiece with a nicotine plug to deliver the nicotine to the mucous membranes of the mouth. The nicotine in the cartridges is released by frequent puffing over 20 minutes. You may use up a cartridge all at once or puff on it for a few minutes at a time until the nicotine is finished. Try different schedules to see what works best for you. If you continue smoking while using nicotine inhalation, you may experience adverse side effects.

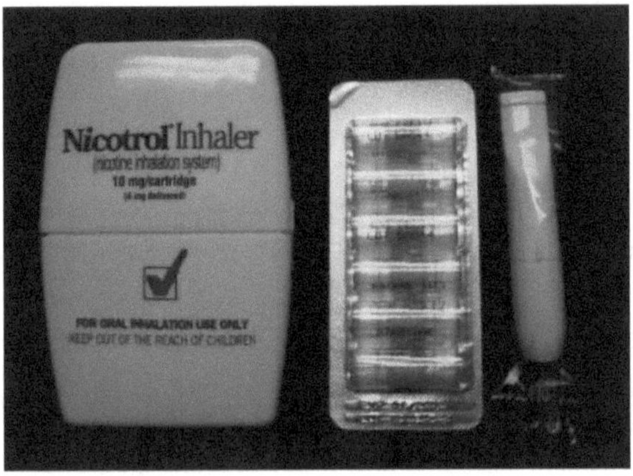


**M A H Russell et al (1983)-**A nasal solution was developed containing 2 mg nicotine for use as a kind of liquid snuff. Its absorption was studied in three subjects. An average peak of plasma nicotine concentrations of 86.9 nmol/l (14.1 ng/ml) was reached seven and a half minutes after taking the solution.This compared with an average peak of 158.4nmol/l (25.7ng/ml) one and a half minutes after completing (but seven and a half minutes after starting) a middle tar cigarette (1-4 mg nicotine) and an average peak of 52-4 nmol/l (8-5 ng/ml) after chewing nicotine gum (2 mg nicotine) for 30 minutes. The more rapid and efficient absorption of nicotine from the nasal nicotine solution than from nicotine chewing gum suggests that it might prove a useful aid to giving up smoking. Nasal nicotine solution might be particularly useful in smokers for whom the gum was less suitable on account of dentures or peptic ulcers or who experience nausea and dyspeptic symptoms from the gum.[93]

**P Tønnesen et al (1983)-**A1-year, randomized, double-blind, placebo-controlled study to evaluate the efficacy of a new nicotine inhaler system for smoking cessation at medical outpatient clinic with physicians experienced in smoking cessation assistance in 286 volunteers who smoked at least 10 cigarettes daily recruited through a local newspaper. Subjects were randomly allocated to nicotine inhalers (n=145) or placebo (n=141) to be used for 3 months followed by tapering for 3 months in the context of minimal levels of advice and support. Continuous smoking abstinence at weeks 6,12, 24, and 52 was verified by measurements of carbon monoxide in expired air. Continuous smoking abstinence was significantly higher for the active nicotine inhaler group compared with the placebo inhaler group. The respective success rates were 28% and 12% after 6 weeks, 21% and 9% after 12 weeks, 17% and 8% after 6 months, and 15% and 5% after 1 year (*P*=.02 to.001). The mean nicotine substitution based on cotinine determinations after 2 weeks was 43% (SD-45%) of smoking levels. The treatment was well tolerated, and no serious adverse events were reported. In this setting the nicotine inhaler appeared safe to use and increased success rates of smoking cessation attempts.[94]

**Karl O Fagerström et al (2000)-**A study was conducted to monitor the effect of a novel nicotine delivery device that may produce fewer carcinogens (Eclipse) on cigarette smoking, carbon monoxide and nicotine concentrations, and motivation to give up smoking. The smoker's own brand of cigarette and a nicotine replacement product (Nicotrol inhaler) were used as comparisons. After baseline data, smokers were randomised to either Eclipse or inhaler for two weeks and then switched to the other product for another two weeks. Thereafter a second baseline was obtained. Fifty smokers were included and data are reported for the 40 with complete data sets. The smokers were not trying to quit but were interested in trying a new product to reduce their risk. They visited a smoking clinic 10 times during the six week period of the trial. Counselling was not given. A teach visit smoking status and carbon monoxide concentrations were recorded. In half of the visits withdrawal symptoms, attitudes towards smoking, heart rate, and blood nicotine concentrations were also recorded. Eclipse use decreased the number of cigarettes smoked per day (cpd) from 19.1 cpd at baseline to 2.1 cpd ($p < 0.001$), but increased carbon monoxide concentrations in parts per million (ppm) from21.0 ppm to 33.0 ppm ($p < 0.001$). A similar decrease in cigarettes smoked per day was seen with the Nicotrol inhaler, from 19.1 cpd to 4.8 cpd ($p < 0.001$), but carbon monoxide decreased from 21.0 ppm to 12.7 ppm ($p < 0.001$). The blood nicotine concentration remained fairly stable with Eclipse, increasing slightly from 16.8 ng/ml to 18.0 ng/ml, while for the inhaler a significant drop was noted, from 16.8 ng/ ml to 12.2 ng/ml ($p < 0.002$). Few significant adverse events occurred with Eclipse. Eclipse can dramatically decrease cigarette consumption without causing withdrawal symptoms or decreases in nicotine concentrations or motivation to quit altogether. Unlike the inhaler, Eclipse produces an increase in carbon monoxide concentration so it may not be a safer cigarette.[95]

**Abraham Bohadana et al (2000)-**A double-blind, randomized, placebo- controlled trial was conducted to comparethe efficacy of the nicotine inhaler plus nicotine patch vs nicotine inhaler plus placebo patch for smoking cessation in 400 subjects who had smoked 10 or more cigarettes per day for 3 years or longer. Group 1 (n=200) received the nicotine inhaler plus nicotine patch (delivering 15 mg of nicotine per 16 hours) for 6 weeks, then inhaler plus placebo patch for 6 weeks, then inhaler alone for 14 weeks. Group 2 (n=200) received the nicotine inhaler plus placebo patch for 12 weeks, then inhaler for 14 weeks. Inhaler was used at a rate of 6 to 12 cartridges per day ad libitum for 3 months and then tapered off. Main outcome measures were complete abstinence (self-reported) and expired carbon dioxide concentration less than 10 ppm. Group 1 vs group 2 complete abstinence rates were 60.5% and 47.5% at 6 weeks ($P$=.009), 42.0% and 31.0% at 12 weeks ($P$=.02), 25.0% and 22.5% at 6 months ($P$=.56), and 19.5% and 14.0% at 12 months ($P$=.14). One-year survival analysis showed a significant association between abstinence and treatment with nicotine inhaler plus nicotine patch ($P$=.04). Mean nicotine substitution at week 6was 60.1% (group 1) and 24.6% (group 2) ($P$<.001). At 12 months, the frequency of respiratory symptoms in abstinent subjects fell significantly and lung function showed a trend toward improvement.The most common adverse events were throat irritation (inhaler) and itching (patch). Treatment with the nicotine inhaler plus nicotine patch resulted in significantly higher cessation rates than inhaler plus placebo patch.[96]

**S Hand et al (2002)-**A randomised trial was conducted to determine effectiveness of nicotine replacement therapy (NRT) in hospital patient referred by their hospital doctor to the smoking cessation counsellor and who agreed to participate to receive either NRT given as a nicotine patch daily and a nicotine inhalator on an as needed basis plus advice and support (AS+NRT), or to receive just advice and support (AS). Claims of smoking cessation were validated at 1 week, 3 months, 6 months, and 1 year by carbon monoxide (CO) breath testing. A total of 245 patients were randomised, 136 AS+NRT and 109 AS. There were no significant demographic differences between the two groups at baseline. At 1 year 35 (14%) had sustained cessation confirmed by a CO breath test, 20/136 (15%) AS+NRT and 15/109 (14%) AS, p=0.857. One hundred and ten patients gave up smoking for at least 1 week, 54% AS+NRT and 33% AS ($p<0.001$). By 6 months there was no significant difference between the two groups (22/136 (16%) AS+NRT and 15/109 (14%) AS). In hospital patients NRT, given as regular daily patches plus an inhalator to be used as needed, did not add to the smoking cessation rate achieved at 1 year by regular advice and support, despite significantly increasing the cessation rate at 1 week.[97]

**Eva Kralikova et al (2009)-**A multi-centre, double-blind placebo-controlled study evaluated the efficacy and safety of nicotine 4 mg gum or nicotine 10 mg inhaler inhelping smokers (N = 314) to reduce or quit smoking. It included smokers willing to control their smoking, and participants could set individual goals, to reduce or quit. The study was placebo-controlled, randomized in a ratio of 2:1 (Active: Placebo), and subjects could choose inhaler or gum after randomization. Outcome was short-term (from Week 6 to Month 4) and long-term (from Month 6 to Month 12) abstinence or reduction. Abstinence was defined as not a single cigarette smoked and expired CO readings of <10 ppm. Smoking reduction was defined as a reduction in number of cigarettes per day by 50% or more versus baseline, verified by a lower-than-baseline CO reading at each visit during the same periods. Significantly more smokers managed to quit in the Active group than in the Placebo group. Sustained abstinence rates at 4 months were 42/209 (20.1%) subjects in the Active group and 9/105 (8.6%) subjects in the Placebo group ($p$=0.009).

Sustained abstinence rates at 12 months were 39/209 (18.7%) and 9/105 (8.6%), respectively ($p = 0.019$). Smoking reduction did not differ between the groups, either at short-term or long-term. Twelve-month reduction results were 17.2% vs. 18.1%, respectively. No serious adverse events were reported. Treatment with 10 mg nicotine inhaler or 4 mg nicotine chewing gum resulted in a significantly higher abstinence rate than placebo. In addition a large number of smokers managed to reduce their cigarette consumption by more than 50% compared to baseline.[98]

### 3.4.E. NICOTINE SPRAY:

Nicotine nasal spray comes as a liquid to spray into the nose. It should be used along with a smoking cessation program, which may include a support group, counselling, or specific cognitive or behavioural techniques. It allows smokers to cut back on their intake of nicotine gradually. Nicotine is absorbed rapidly through the nasal membranes.

**Directions**

1. Wash your hands.
2. Gently blow your nose to clear your nasal passages.
3. Remove the cap of the nasal spray by pressing in the circles on the side of the bottle.
4. To prime the pump before the first use, hold the bottle in front of a tissue or paper towel.
5. Pump the spray bottle six to eight times until a fine spray appears. Throw away the tissue or towel.
6. Tilt your head back slightly.
7. Insert the tip of the bottle as far as you comfortably can into one nostril, pointing the tip toward the back of your nose. Breathe through your mouth.
8. Pump the spray firmly and quickly one time. Do not sniff, swallow, or inhale while spraying. If your nose runs, gently sniff to keep the nasal spray in your nose. Wait two or three minutes before blowing your nose.
9. Repeat steps six to eight for the second nostril. Replace the cover on the spray bottle.

If you have not stopped smoking at the end of four weeks, talk with your doctor.

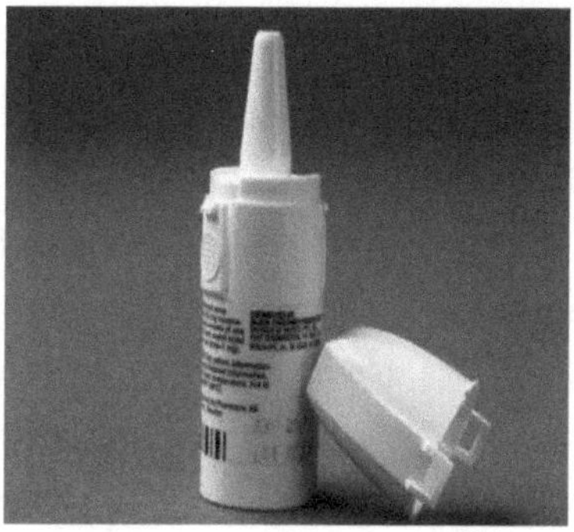

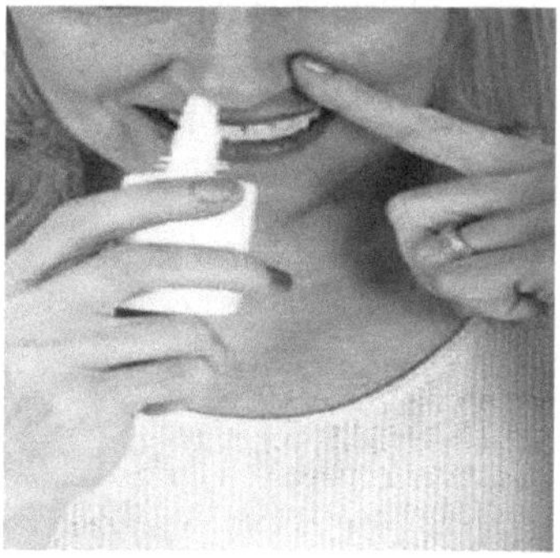

**Peter Hajek et al (1999)-**Randomized trial with assessments was done at Hospital smokers' clinic at the quit date and 1, 4, and 12 weeks later to provide a basis for rational advice by comparing nicotine gum, a transdermal patch, nasal spray, and an inhaler. Male and female community volunteers (N = 504) smoking 10 or more cigarettes per day and seeking help to stop smoking. Patients were given brief advice, and purchased their nicotine replacement treatment at approximately half the regular retail price. Nicotine replacement treatment use, ratings of withdrawal symptoms, ratings of product characteristics and helpfulness, and biochemically validated continuous lapse-free abstinence were main outcome measures. The products did not differ in their effects on withdrawal discomfort, urges to smoke, or rates of abstinence. The continuous validated 12-week abstinence rates were 20%, 21%, 24%, and 24% in the gum, patch, spray, and inhaler groups, respectively. Compliance with recommended nicotine replacement treatment use was high for the patch, low for gum, and very low for the spray and the inhaler. The spray was underused because of adverse effects more often than the other products. The inhaler was rated as more embarrassing to use than the other products, but provided at least as much nicotine as the gum. When asked about nicotine replacement treatment products available, physicians should note that, despite low compliance with the recommended dose of the spray and inhaler and differences in product ratings, overall, there are no notable differences between the products in their effects on withdrawal discomfort, perceived helpfulness, or general efficacy.[99]

**Mark L. Rubinstein et al (2008)-**A randomized, open-label, 12-week trial was conducted to determine the feasibility and utility of using nicotine nasal spray (NNS) in adolescent smokers who want to quit smoking. Forty adolescent smokers between 15 and 18 years-old, who smoked 5 or more cigarettes daily for at least 6 months were recruited from several San Francisco Bay area schools from 2005–2007 and were assigned to receive either weekly counselling alone (control) for 8 weeks or 8 weeks of counselling alongwith 6 weeks of NNS. Self-reported smoking abstinence verified by both expired-air carbon monoxide and salivary cotinine. There was no difference in cessation rates, the numbers of cigarettes smoked per day or cotinine levels at 12 weeks ($p$=.16, $p$=.22, and $p$=.16 respectively). Fifty seven percent of participants stopped using their spray after only one week. The most commonly reported side effect was nasal irritation and burning (34.8%) followed by complaints about the taste and smell (13%).The unpleasant side effects, poor adherence, and consequent lack of efficacy observed in this pilot study did not support the use of nicotine nasal spray as an adjunct to counselling for adolescent smokers wishing to quit.[100]

__Rey et al (2009)-__Randomized, open, controlled trial included 50 patients who were heavy smokers, willing to quit, and attending an academic outpatient clinic in Western Switzerland was conducted to assess the impact of instructional guidance in the regular use of use nicotine nasal spray (NNS) on the true use of NNS during the first three weeks of cessation. Patients were randomized to instruction on NNS use as "ad libitum" (administration whenever cravings appear; control group) or to use NNS when craving appears and at least every hour when awake (intervention group). Intakes were monitored using an electronic device fixed in the spray unit (MDILog™) during the first three weeks of use. Self reported abstinence from smoking at six months was confirmed by expired-air carbon monoxide. One patient was lost to follow-up. At baseline randomization, the group receiving instruction to use NNS hourly included more women, patients with previous desires to quit, and patients with more psychiatric comorbidities and less somatic complaints compared to the group instructed to use NNS with cravings (group imbalance). Both groups self-administered more than the daily recommended dosage of 8 uses. Mean daily usage was 13.6 dose/day and 11.1 dose/day for the group instructed to use NNS hourly and with cravings, respectively. Adjusting for baseline imbalance, the increased daily doses in the intervention group (hourly use) remained non significant compared to use (-0.5 dose/day; CI 95% -6.2; 5.3, from day 1 to day 7; and 2.3 dose/day; CI 95% -5.4; 10.0, from day 8 to day 21). Instructing patients to use the NNS daily had no effect on smoking cessation at six months (RR = 0.69; CI 95% 0.34; 1.39). Heavy smokers willing to quit use NNS frequently, regardless of the instructions given. Recommending the use of NNS only when craving appeared for heavy smokers willing to quit seems acceptable compared to prescribing hourly administration.[101]

### 3.4.F. NICOTINE LOZENGES

This is a more recent addition to the growing number of tools to combat nicotine withdrawal symptoms.

**Directions**

For weeks one to six of treatment, you should use one lozenge every one to two hours.Use at least nine lozenges per day to increase your chances of quitting. During week seven to nine, you should use one lozenge every two to four hours. Weeks 10 to 12, you should use one lozenge every four to eight hours. Do not use more than five lozenges in six hours or more than 20 lozenges per day. Do not use more than one lozenge at a time or use one lozenge right after another. Using too many lozenges at a time or one after another can cause side effects such as hiccups, heartburn, and nausea. Do not eat while the lozenge is in your mouth. Stop usingthe nicotine lozenges after 12 weeks. After 12 weeks if you still feel the need to use nicotine lozenges, talk to your doctor.

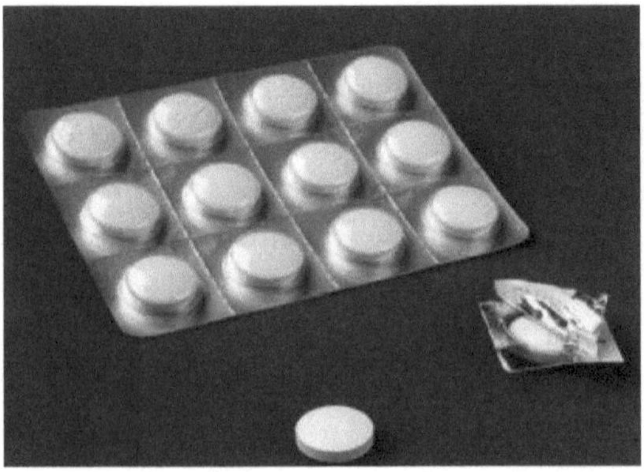

**Saul Shiffman et al (2002)-**A Double-blind, placebo-controlled, randomized clinical trial with parallel arms study tested the safety and efficacy of a new nicotine polacrilex (2- and 4-mg nicotine lozenges) for smoking cessation. Smokers (n = 1818) were assigned to a lozenge dose on the basis of nicotine dependence, assessed by time to the first cigarette of the day. Low-dependence smokers were randomized to receive the 2-mg nicotine (n =459) or placebo (n = 458) lozenge; high-dependence smokers, the 4-mg nicotine (n = 450) or placebo (n = 451) lozenge. They assessed abstinence at 6, 12, 24, and 52 weeks and analyzed craving and withdrawal symptoms. Treatment with the nicotine lozenge resulted in significantly greater 28-day abstinence at 6 weeks, for the 2-mg (46.0% vs. 29.7%; odds ratio [OR], 2.10; 95% confidence interval [CI], 1.59-2.79; P<.001) and the 4-mg(48.7% vs. 20.8%; OR, 3.69; 95% CI, 2.74-4.96; P<.001) lozenges, compared with placebo. Smokers who used more lozenges achieved significantly better treatment effects. Use of the active lozenge also resulted in reduced craving and withdrawal. Most adverse events were moderate and resembled those seen with nicotine gum. The nicotine lozenge was a safe and effective new treatment for smoking cessation in low- and high-dependence smokers.[102]

**Jon O. Ebbert et al (2010)-**A study was done to evaluate a reduction approach in smokeless tobacco (ST) users. They conducted an open-label pilot study to determine if the 4-mg nicotine lozenge with a behavioral intervention could facilitate ST use reduction compared with a behavioral intervention alone. Eligible subjects were ST users not interested in quitting. One hundred and two subjects were randomized. Both interventions were associated with significant decreases in ST use and toxicant exposure and with increased abstinence, quit attempts, and duration of abstinence. However, no significant differences were observed between groups for these outcomes. A behavioral intervention with or without the nicotine lozenge might be effective for decreasing both ST use and toxicant exposure and for increasing tobacco abstinence, quit attempts, and duration of abstinence. The use of reduction strategies for ST users not interested in quitting deserves further evaluation as an intervention strategy.[103]

**Robert A. Schnoll et al (2010)-**A randomized, open-label effectiveness trial was conducted at twelve medical sites participating in the National Cancer Institute's Community Clinical Oncology Program to compare the effectiveness of transdermal nicotine vs. nicotine lozenge for smoking cessation and identified predictors of treatment response. The sample consisted of 642 treatment-seeking smokers randomized to twelve weeks of transdermal nicotine or nicotine lozenge. Smoker characteristics were assessed at baseline, and 24-hour point prevalence abstinence confirmed with breath carbon monoxide (CO) was evaluated at end of treatment (EOT) and at a 6- month follow-up. There was a trend for higher quit rates for transdermal nicotine vs. nicotine lozenge at EOT (24.3% vs. 18.7%, p = .10) and 6-months (15.6% vs. 10.9%, p = .10). A logistic regression model of EOT quit rates showed smokers who preferred transdermal nicotine, were not reactive to smoking cues, and did not use nicotine to alleviate distress or stimulate cognitive function had higher quit rates on transdermal nicotine. A logistic regression model of 6-month quit rates showed smokers who preferred transdermal nicotine had higher quit rates on transdermal nicotine, and smokers who used nicotine to alleviate distress or stimulate cognitive processes had lower quit rates on nicotine lozenge. Transdermal nicotine may be more effective than nicotine lozenge for smokers who prefer transdermal nicotine and do not smoke to alleviate emotional distress or stimulate cognitive function. [104]

## NON-NICOTINE REPLACEMENT THERAPIES

**AWilson et al (2006)-**Patient questionnaire survey was conducted to examine the context in which nicotine replacement therapy (NRT) and bupropion are prescribed in UK general practice and whether guidelines are being followed at 25 general practices from the Trent Focus Collaborative Research Network in South Yorkshire and East Midlands, UK. Participating practices posted a questionnaire to up to 40 patients prescribed NRT and bupropion respectively in the previous 3–9 months. The response rate for people prescribed NRT was 44.7% (323/723) and for bupropion 42.5% (77/181). Patients reported initiating the prescription request in 258 cases (65%), whereas GPs were reported as suggesting it in 49 (12%), smoking cessation services (SCS) in 38 (10%), and practice nurses in 36 (9%).Of those who could recall the content of the consultation in which NRT or bupropion was prescribed, 191 (79%) reported receiving advice on treatment use and 209 (68%) were encouraged to set a quit date. Follow up by SCS was recommended to186 (64%) and practice follow up was offered to 212 (63%), but 41 (15%) reported no offer of follow up support. The majority of patients reported receiving advice and follow up in line with guidelines. However, relatively few prescriptions were not suggested by GPs or practice nurses and, in a significant minority of cases, followed up by the practice nor additional support from SCS was recommended. More active implementation of guidelines could increase the impact of general practice on the prevalence of smoking.[105]

**Florian Vogt et al (2006)-**Two studies were done to observe General practitioners' (GPs) negative beliefs about nicotine dependence medications that might act as barriers to prescribing them. Study1: Twenty-five GPs from 16 practices across London were interviewed in this qualitative study. Framework analysis was used to identify key themes. Study 2: A convenience sample of 367 GPs completed an internet-based survey. Path-analysis was used to examine the relations between beliefs and intentions to prescribe smoking cessation medications. Study 1 showed nicotine replacement therapy (NRT) and bupropion were generally perceived as effective and cost-effective, the effectiveness of NRT was seen as critically dependent on behavioural support for smoking cessation. GPs perceived bupropion as dangerous and were concerned about its side effects. Study 2 showed GPs' beliefs had medium (NRT, $f^2$ = .23) to large (bupropion, $f2$=.45; NRT without support, $f^2$=.59) effects on their intentions to prescribe medications. Beliefs about effectiveness of NRT and bupropion and the perceived danger of bupropion were the key predictors of intentions to prescribe NRT and bupropion, respectively. Beliefs about neglecting psychological aspects of smoking and incorrect use had indirect effects on intentions to prescribe NRT without support. GPs vary in their beliefs about the effectiveness and safety of smoking cessation medications. Their intentions to prescribe these medications vary in line with these beliefs. Interventions aimed at increasing the likelihood with which GPs prescribe these medications might be more effective if they addressed these beliefs.[106]

**BUPROPION:**

Bupropion is also known as Zyban or Wellbutrin. Zyban is the trade name for the medication when it is prescribed for smoking cessation and Wellbutrin is the trade name for the medication when it is prescribed for depression. It is therefore classified as an antidepressant. Bupropion works by blocking the dopamine transporter pump preventing the transport of dopamine back into the neuron, and thereby increasing the amount of dopamine in the synaptic cleft.

Bupropion comes in two forms of tablets to be taken by mouth: a regular tablet and a sustained-release or extended-release (long-acting) tablet. The regular tablet (Wellbutrin) is usually taken three or four times a day, with doses at least six hours apart. The sustained-release tablet (Wellbutrin SR or Zyban) is usually taken once or twice daily in the morning and afternoon. It is contraindicated in seizure disorders, liver disease, anorexia.

**Directions**

- Doctor probably starts a low dose of bupropion and gradually increase the dose over time.
- It may take four weeks or longer before you feel the full benefit of bupropion.
- Continue to take bupropion even if you feel well.
- Your doctor will probably decrease the dose gradually over a period of two weeks prior to stopping the medication.
- If you forget, skip, or miss a dose, then continue your regular dosing schedule. Do not take a double dose to make up for a missed dose.
- Always allow the full scheduled amount of time to pass between doses of bupropion.

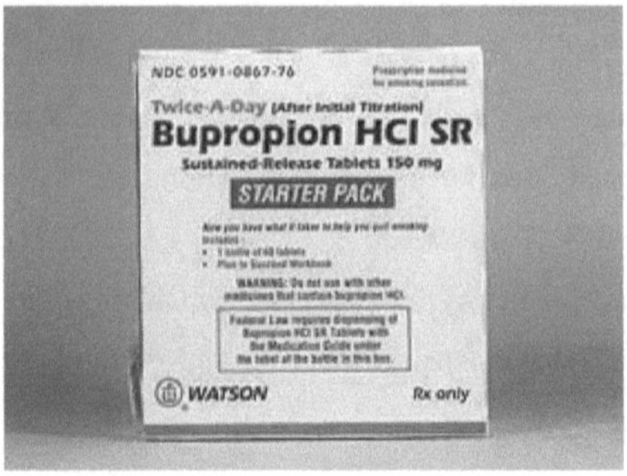


**Richard D. Hurt et al (1997)-**A double-blind study was conducted for placebo-controlled trial of a sustained-release form of bupropion for smoking cessation. The 615 subjects were randomly assigned to receive placebo or bupropion at a dose of 100, 150, or 300 mg per day for seven weeks. The target quitting date was one week after the beginning of treatment. Brief counselling was provided at base line, weekly during treatment, and at 8, 12, 26, and 52 weeks. The rates of smoking cessation were confirmed by carbon monoxide measurements. The rates for the 150-mg group (P-0.02) and the 300-mg group (P-0.01) but not the 100-mg group (P-0.09) were significantly better than those for the placebo group. Among the subjects who were continuously abstinent through the end of treatment, the mean absolute weight gain was inversely associated with the dose (a gain of 2.9 kg in the placebo group, 2.3 kg in 100-mg and 150-mg groups, and 1.5 kg inthe 300 mg group; P-0.02). No effects of treatment were observed on depression scores as measured serially by the Beck Depression Inventory. Thirty-seven subjects stopped treatment prematurely because of adverse events. A sustained-release form of bupropion was effective for smoking cessation and was accompanied by reduced weight gain and minimal side effects. Many participants in all groups were smoking at one year.[107]

**Douglas E. Jorenby et al (1999)-** A double-blind, placebo-controlled comparison of sustained release bupropion (244 subjects), a nicotine patch (244 subjects), bupropion and a nicotine patch (245 subjects), and placebo (160 subjects) for smoking cessation was conducted. Treatment consisted of nine weeks of bupropion (150 mg a day for the first three days, and then 150 mg twice daily) or placebo, as well as eight weeks of nicotine-patch therapy (21 mg per day during weeks 2 through 7, 14 mg per day during week 8, and 7 mg per day during week 9)or placebo.The target day for quitting smoking was usually day 8. The abstinence rates at 12 months were 15.6% in the placebo group, as compared with 16.4 % in the nicotine-patch group, 30.3 % in the bupropion group (P<0.001), and 35.5% in the group given bupropion and the nicotine patch (P<0.001). By week 7, subjects in the placebo group had gained an average of 2.1kg, as compared with again of 1.6 kg in the nicotine-patch group, again of 1.7 kg in the bupropion group, and again of 1.1 kg in the combined-treatment group (P<0.05). Weight gain at seven weeks was significantly less in the combined-treatment group than in the bupropion group and the placebo group (P<0.05 for both comparisons). A total of 311 subjects (34.8 percent) discontinued one or both medications. Seventy-nine subjects stopped treatment because of adverse events: 6 in the placebo group (3.8%), 16 in the nicotine-patch group (6.6 %), 29 in the bupropion group (11.9 %), and 28 in the combined treatment group (11.4 %). The most common adverse events were insomnia and headache. Abstinence rates were higher with combination therapy than with bupropion alone, but the difference was not statistically significant.[108]

**Andy McEwen et al (2001)-**A study assessed English General Practitioners'(GPs) attitudes towards reimbursement of NRT and bupropion. Postal survey of a randomly selected national sample of GPs; 376 GPs completed the questionnaire after one reminder; effective response rate: 53%. There was no difference between the responses of GPs who responded to the initial request and those who responded only after a reminder suggesting minimal bias due to non-response. Forty-three percent thought that bupropion should not be on NHS prescription while 42% thought that it should be (15% did not know); Fifty percent thought that NRT should not be on National health survey (NHS) prescription while 42% thought it should be (8% did not know). A principal components analysis of responses to the individual questions on NRT and bupropion revealed that GPs' attitudes could be understood in terms of a single 'pro-con' dimension accounting for 53% of the total variance which made no distinction between the two medications. GPs in England appear to be divided in their attitudes to medications to aid smoking cessation and appear not to discriminate in their views between different types of medication or different aspects of their use. It suggested that their attitudes were generated by quite fundamental values. Addressing these values might be important in encouraging GPs to adhere more closely to national and international guidelines.[109]

**F Antonanzas et al (2003)-**A study was conducted to assess the efficiency of three smoking cessation strategies based on pharmacotherapies in Spain included a mixture of primary care physician advice, group therapy and will power, combined with the use of drugs in a small proportion of individuals. A cost-effectiveness evaluation was used to calculate the cost per death prevented and per year of life saved in each scenario. The analysis used a time horizon of 20 years and was based on an adaptation of the HECOS model, sponsored by WHO-Euro, which enables comparison of distinct pharmacotherapy interventions. Epidemiological data were based on the National Health Survey (1997) and the National Institute of Statistics (1999). The cost-effectiveness ratio of bupropion at 5 years was 70,939 euros per death prevented and was 37,305 euros per year of life saved. When the time horizon was increased to 20 years, these figures became net savings of 28,166 and 3,265 euros, respectively. The cost-effectiveness ratios for both nicotine gums and patches were higher than that for bupropion: 171,834 euros per death prevented at 5 years and 90,362 euros per year of life saved for patches and 513,004 euros per death prevented and 269,772 euros per year of life saved at 5 years. Bupropion treatment for 1 year would prevent a greater number of deaths than the alternative strategies due to the decrease in the number of smokers. The cost of some tobacco cessation methods, such as primarycare physician advice and group therapy, was low but their efficacy was also low. When assessing interventions and their costs economic evaluation shows that in the long run greater use of bupropion generates net savings in tobacco-related health costs.[110]

**Joel A. Simon et al (2004)-**In an outpatient randomized blinded smoking cessation trial, conducted at the San Francisco Veterans Affairs Medical Center, a total of 244 current smokers were enrolled. Among them 121 received a 7-week course of bupropion and 123 received placebos. All participants received 2 months of transdermal nicotine replacement therapy and 3 months of cognitive-behavioural counselling. They determined on-medication treatment, end-of-medication treatment, 3-month, 6-month, and 1-year quit rates.During treatment with bupropion vs placebo, there was a trend toward increased quit rates among participants randomized to bupropion; the self-reported end of- medication treatment quit rates were 64% for the bupropion group vs 57% for the placebo group ($P$=.23). The trend favouring bupropion persisted at 3 months of follow- up ($P$=.12) but was not apparent at 6 months and 1 year of follow-up (both $P$=.78). The 12-month quit rates, validated by either saliva cotinine or spousal proxy, were 22% in the bupropion group and 28% in the placebo group ($P$=.31). Based on biochemical validation, 19% of the bupropion group vs 24% of the placebo group had quit smoking by 1 year ($P$=.36). In this randomized blinded trial of mostly veteran participants, the addition of a brief 7-week bupropion trial to treatment with nicotine replacement therapy and counselling did not significantly increase smoking cessation rates.[111]

**Kristian Bolin et al (2006)-**A Study was conducted to calculate incremental cost-utility ratios (cost per quality-adjusted life-year [QALY] gained) for bupropion (Zyban; GlaxoSmithKline; Sweden), as compared to nicotine replacement therapy (NRT) in smoking cessation programs for a follow-up period of 20 years. The Global Health Outcomes simulation model was used for a male cohort and for a female cohort as a point of departure but was further extended in order to include the following: (1) the indirect effects of smoking cessation on production and consumption in the economy, and (2) morbidity-specific QALYs gained. Model cohort was consisting of 612,851 male and 780,970 female smokers, distributed by age, >35 years old, as in the Swedish population of 2001. Bupropion, as compared to NRT (nicotine patches and nicotine gums), in smoking cessation programs for a follow-up period of 20 years. When the indirect effects on production and consumption were taken into account, bupropion was cost saving in comparison to both NRTs. When only the direct costs were included, bupropion was still cost saving in comparison to nicotine gum. The incremental costs per QALY gained were relatively low for bupropion in comparison to nicotine patches, 6,600 Swedish kronas (SEK) (approximately €725) per QALY gained for men and 4,900 SEK (approximately € 535) for women, all calculations in 2001 Swedish prices. Results were, however, more sensitive to quit rates and intervention costs than to other variables. Bupropion is a cost-effective therapy in smoking cessation programs. Further studies reported even higher effectiveness in terms of quit rates than was assumed here.[112]

**Melanie Y Bertram et al (2006)-**A cost-effectiveness analysis using a deterministic Markov model, and cost per disability-adjusted life year (DALY) averted over a lifetimeas the outcome measure was done to estimate the cost-effectiveness of bupropion and NRT, and the potential financial impact of public reimbursement of NRT in Australia in current smokers, motivated to quit, in Australia in 2000. They conducted three interventions-(1) NRT; (2) bupropion; and (3) a combined strategy using bupropion as the first-line treatment and NRTin those who fail to quit smoking or have adverse reactions to bupropion. Results showed Quitting smoking could increase life expectancy of current smokers by 1–7.6 years depending on age at cessation and sex. Providing bupropion to current smokers who were motivated to quit would cost A$7900 (95% uncertainty interval A$6000 to A$10 500) for each DALY averted; NRT patches would cost A$17 000 (A$9000 to A$28 000) for each DALY averted, with similar results even if used as a second-line treatment following initial failure to quit using bupropion. If 6% of current smokers were to use NRT following inclusion on the Pharmaceutical Benefits Scheme (PBS), this would result in an annual cost of A $40–110 million to the PBS depending on the listed price. Compared with other drugs included on the PBS, bupropion and NRT are both highly cost-effective smoking cessation interventions, and including NRT on the PBS would have a moderate financial impact.Given the size able health burden of smoking, and the large individual benefits of quitting smoking, increasing the availability of alternative aids and uptake of these strategies through public reimbursement would be a positive and rational step towards further reducing tobacco-related disease burden in Australia andother countries where NRT was currently not subsidised.[113]

**A. Paula Cupertino et al (2008)-**A population-based clinical trial identified 750 smokers in primary care practices and independent of their stage of change offered them a free treatment course of either bupropion or transdermal nicotine replacement (TNR). Smokers opting for pharmacotherapy completed standardized contraindication screens that were reviewed by the patient's primary care physician. Most participants (67%) requested pharmacotherapy. Use of pharmacotherapy was positively associated with higher nicotine dependence and readiness to quit. Of the smokers requesting pharmacotherapy, 51% requested bupropion and 49% requested TNR. Choice of bupropion was related to no history of heart disease and no previous use of bupropion. Although potential contraindications to treatments were identified for 21.7% of bupropion and 6.6% or TNR recipients, physicians rarely felt that these potential contraindications precluded the use of these agents. When cost was removed as a barrier, a large proportion of rural smokers were eager to use smoking cessation pharmacotherapy, especially agents that they had not tried before. Although some comorbid conditions and concurrent drug therapies were considered contraindications, particularly to bupropion, physicians rarely considered these clinically significant risks enough to deny pharmacotherapy.[114]

**Jennifer W. Tidey & Damaris J. Rohsenow (2009)-**A laboratory study examined the effects of 300 mg/day bupropion, compared with placebo, on baseline and smoking cue-elicited urge to smoke and other measures in smokers who stated that they did ( *n* = 8) or did not ( *n* =17) intend to quit smoking within 6 months. Significant interactions indicated that bupropion reduced the effects of acute abstinence on smoking urges in the presence of neutral cues, only in those who intended to quit. Bupropion and intention to quit did not reduce the effects of acute abstinence on urges in the presence of smoking cues and did not reduce nicotine withdrawal symptoms or smoking behaviour between sessions. This study was one of the first placebo-controlled examinations of the effects of bupropion on cue reactivity and provides support for the idea that laboratory smoking studies might be more likely to detect effects of pharmacological treatments for smoking when they enrolled smokers who intended to quit.[115]

**Andy McEwen et al (2009)-**A study was done to directly compare of the short-term validated abstinence rates of NRT and bupropion in a clinical setting. Data were routinely collected from 2626 clients setting a quit date (82% of those registering) with two London NHS Stop Smoking Services that offered behavioural support combined with pharmacotherapy (NRT and bupropion). Contrary to what would be expected from multiple randomized controlled trials, the CO-validated 3–4 week abstinence rate in clients using NRT was higher than for bupropion (42% versus 34%, p = .003). This difference persisted even when controlling for smoking characteristics, demographic variables and treatment variables 1.40 (95% CI = 1.08 – 1.83). Given that the level of behavioural support received by clients on each medication was identical, the most plausible explanation for the difference in effectiveness between NRT and bupropion perhaps lies with how clients of the Stop Smoking Services obtained their medications. ObtainingNRT was relatively easy for clients throughout the study period whilst this was not the case for bupropion. This study suggested that implementation issues and/or self-selection might influence the effectiveness of medications in health care, as opposed to research, settings.[116]

**M. Al-haj (2004)-**A piloted questionnaire study was done in 57 bupropion clients to evaluate the clinical use of bupropion (Zyban) as an aid for smoking cessation in the first year post-marketing in Bradford area,United Kingdom. The result showed that 63% of participants had given up smoking after treatment.Family advice and support significantly enhanced the cessation rate with Bupropion treatment. The most commonly reported adverse effects were insomnia, headache and dry mouth. It was concluded that sustained released Bupropion is an effective aid for smoking cessation which was well tolerated by the respondents.[117]

## VARENICLINE

It was developed by Pfizer through modifying the structure of cytisine, Its trade name Chantix, is the most recent medication that is FDA approved to treat smoking addiction. It is available by prescription only. Currently there is no generic form. Varenicline is a partial agonist to a subtype of the nicotinic acetylcholine receptor. A partial agonist is a compound that both stimulates and inhibits the receptor to a mild degree, thereby eliminating any withdrawal effects associated with smoking cessation, but also eliminating the possibility of deriving any additional pleasure from smoking. It therefore acts like a thermostat, stimulating the receptor when nicotine levels are low and blocking the receptor when nicotine levels are high.

Varenicline was fast tracked by the U.S. Food and Drug Administration in February 2006, shortening its approval from 10 to 6 months because of its demonstrated effectiveness in clinical trials and perceived lack of safety issues. The FDA approved varenicline on May 11, 2006, which became available in the U.S. public August 1, 2006, and in the European Union September 29, 2006.

**Directions**

- Doctor will probably start you on a low dose of varenicline and gradually increase the dose over the first week of treatment.
- Set a quit date to stop smoking, and start taking varenicline one week before that date. You may continue to smoke during this first week, but stop smoking on the quit date. It may take several weeks for you to feel the full benefit of varenicline.
- You may slip and smoke during your treatment. If this happens, you will still be able to stop smoking.
- Continue to take varenicline for 12 weeks.
- If you have completely stopped smoking at the end of the 12 weeks, your doctor may tell you to take varenicline for another 12 weeks. Continuing to take varenicline may ensure that you will not start to smoke again.
- Once you have stopped smoking, your doctor may need to change the doses of some of your other medications.
- If you have not stopped smoking at the end of 12 weeks, tell your doctor so he or she can help you to understand why you were not able to stop smoking and make plans for you to try to quit again.

- Do not use varenicline with other smoking cessation products.
- *If you forget a dose:* Take the missed dose as soon as you remember it. However, if it is almost time for the next dose, skip the missed dose and continue your regular dosing schedule. Do not take a double dose to make up for the missed one.
- Do NOT drink alcohol while taking this medication.

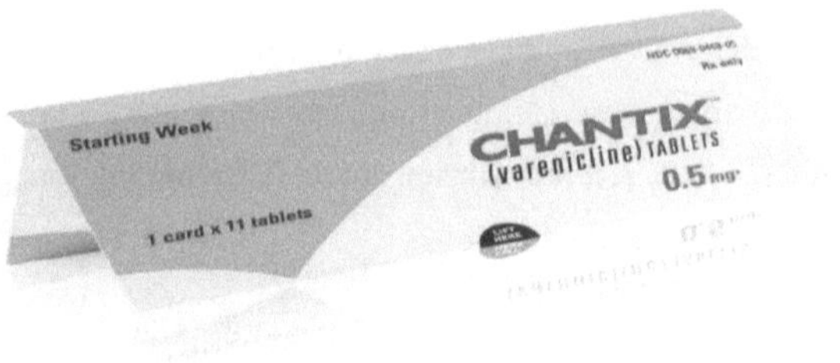


**H-J Aubin et al (2008)-**A 52-week, open-label, randomised, multicentre, phase 3 trial was conducted in Belgium, France, Netherlands, UK and USA to compare a 12-week standard regimen of varenicline with a 10-week standard regimen of transdermal nicotine replacement therapy for smoking cessation. Total of 376 and 370 participants were randomly assigned (1:1) to receive varenicline up titrated to 1 mg twice daily for 12 weeks or transdermal NRT (21 mg/day reducing to 7 mg/day) for 10 weeks respectively. Non-treatment follow up continued to week 52. The primary outcome was the biochemically confirmed (exhaled carbon monoxide (10 ppm) self-reported continuous abstinence rate (CAR) for the last 4 weeks of the treatment period in participants who had taken at least one dose of treatment. Secondary outcomes included CAR from the last 4 weeks of treatment through weeks 24 and 52, and measures of craving, withdrawal and smoking satisfaction. The CAR for the last 4 weeks of treatment was significantly greater for varenicline (55.9%) than NRT (43.2%; OR 1.70, 95% CI 1.26 to 2.28, p=0.001). The week 52 CAR (NRT, weeks 8–52; varenicline, weeks 9–52) was 26.1% for varenicline and 20.3% for NRT (OR 1.40, 95% CI 0.99 to 1.99, p=0.056). Varenicline significantly reduced craving (p=0.001), withdrawal symptoms (p=0.001) and smoking satisfaction (p=0.001) compared with NRT. The most frequent adverse event was nausea (varenicline, 37.2%; NRT, 9.7%).The outcomes of this trial established that abstinence from smoking was greater and craving, withdrawal symptoms and smoking satisfaction were less at the end of treatment with varenicline than with transdermal NRT.[118]

**J Fernández de Bobadilla Osorio et al (2008)-**A study was conducted to analyse the efficiency of varenicline compared with bupropion, NRT (nicotine replacement therapy) and no pharmacological treatment in Spain. A Markov model was developed to analyse the health and economic consequences of smoking cessation therapies. The transition probabilities were taken from published studies. The model allows cost effectiveness analyses for different time frames (10 years, 20 years and life time). Outcomes are measured in terms of incremental life years gained (LYG) and QALYs. Pharmacological costs and costs of medical visits with varenicline and bupropion were considered. Treatment costs of smoking associated morbidity were taken from Spanish studies. The analyses were done under the perspective of the National Health System, discounting costs and health benefits at 3%.The life time cost-effectiveness analysis showed that varenicline dominates all other smoking cessation interventions (more effective at a lower cost). This was due to the higher efficacy of varenicline associated with a reduction in smoking related morbid mortality, which, in the long term, accounts for health care cost savings that overcome the extra cost of varenicline. Varenicline was a dominant and cost effective option compared with all other smoking cessation treatments when the time frame was the life span of the patient.[119]

**Thomas J. Moore et al (2011)-**Two treatments for smoking cessation—varenicline and bupropion—carry Boxed Warnings from the U.S. Food and Drug Administration (FDA) about suicidal/self-injurious behaviour and depression.From the FDA's Adverse Event Reporting System (AERS) database from 1998 through September 2010they selected domestic, serious case reports for varenicline (n=9,575), bupropion for smoking cessation (n = 1,751), and nicotine replacement products (n = 1,917). A composite end point of suicidal/self-injurious behaviour or depression was defined as a case with one or more Preferred Terms in Standardized MedDRA Query (SMQ) for those adverse effects. The main outcome measure was the ratio of reported suicide/self-injuryor depression cases for each drug compared to all other serious events for that drug. Overall they identified 3,249 reported cases of suicidal/self-injurious behavior or depression, 2,925 (90%) for varenicline, 229 (7%) for bupropion, and 95 (3%) for nicotine replacement. Compared to nicotine replacement, the disproportionality results (OR (95% CI)) were varenicline 8.4 (6.8–10.4), and bupropion 2.9 (2.3–3.7). The disproportionality persisted after excluding reports indicating concomitant therapy with any of 58 drugs with suicidal behaviour warnings or precautions in the prescribing information. Varenicline shows a substantial, statistically significant increased risk of reported depression and suicidal/self injurious behaviuor. Bupropion for smoking cessation had smaller increased risks. The findings for varenicline, combined with other problems with its safety profile, render it unsuitable for first-line use in smoking cessation.[120]

**OTHERS**

A number of other medications have been studied, but only two are currently recommended as second-line therapies, should individuals either fail the first-line therapies or experience side effects that contraindicate future use. Second-line therapies are generally used when first-line therapies are contraindicated or some other compelling clinical reason suggests their trial over a first-line therapy.

These other treatments have been evaluated, but the results are inconclusive: - e.g. Appetite suppressants, benzodiazepines, beta-blockers, buspirone, caffeine/ephedrine, cimetidine, dextrose tablets (food supplement), lobeline, moclobemide (monoamine oxidase inhibitor), selective serotonin reuptake inhibitors (SSRIs), such as fluoxetine, paroxetine, citalopram, etc., and naltrexone (ReVia).

Two medications that have proven to be effective as second- line therapies include the tricyclic antidepressant, nortriptyline (trade name, Pamelor), and the antihypertensive, clonidine.

- Nortriptyline blocks the transporter pump and prevents the reuptake of norepinephrine, thus increasing levels of this neurotransmitter in the brain. Norepinephrine release is stimulated by nicotine, so that nortriptyline may aid as an indirect replacement therapy through this action.
- Clonidine is a more complicated medication. It generally reduces what is called sympathetic tone—that is, it reduces the "fight or flight response" by reducing the release of norepinephrine. Clonidine is used not only to reduce blood pressure, but also to treat neuropsychiatric conditions such as Tourette"s disorder and ADHD (attention deficit hyperactivity disorder). It is also used to reduce the effects of opiate withdrawal in opiate-dependent patients.

**Stephanie S. O'Malley et al (2006)-**Six-week double-blind placebo-controlled trial with follow-up was done in an outpatient research center. 400 individuals who smoked 20 or more cigarettes daily were randomly assigned to treatment for 6 weeks with a 21-mg nicotine patch and oral naltrexone hydrochloride (0, 25, 50, or 100 mg/d) after equal random treatment assignment and followed up for 1 year after randomization. The a prior specified primary end points were prolonged 4-week cigarette abstinence after a 2-week grace period in the intent-to-treat sample and weight gain in these abstainers. They found no significant differences in prolonged 4-week abstinence (*P*=.49) or 6-week continuous abstinence after the quit date (*P*=.12) during treatment in the intent-to-treat analysis. Among 295 treatment completers, the 100-mg dose was associated with higher continuous abstinence rates (71.6%) compared with placebo (48%) (odds ratio, 2.73; 95% confidence interval, 1.39-5.39; *P*< 0.01). Among continuous abstainers, the 25-mg naltrexone hydrochloride group gained significantly less weight (mean±SEM, 0.7±0.31 kg) than the placebo group (mean±SEM, 1.9±0.33 kg; *P*_.01). Similar naltrexone dose effects on weight were found for those with prolonged abstinence and treatment completers, irrespective of abstinence. The 100-mg dose of naltrexone hydrochloride appears the most promising for augmenting the efficacy of the nicotine patch on smoking cessation outcomes but requires further study. The significant weight reduction with low-dose naltrexone therapy suggested that it might be useful as a second-line treatment for weight concerned smokers.[121]

**Witold Zatonski et al (2006)-**An uncontrolled, open-label trial sought to obtain an estimate of the 12-month continuous abstinence rates of smokers using cytosine (Tabex) with minimal behavioural support at a smokers" clinic in an oncology centre in Warsaw, Poland. 436 consecutive attendees of the smokers "clinic of whom 191 were male were the subjects .The mean dependence score (Fagerstrom Test for Nicotine Dependence) was 6.1. The standard regimen of Tabex (cytisine) was used, involving 25 days of treatment with minimal behavioural support. Main outcome measure was Self-reported continuous abstinence for 12 months; with abstinence verified by carbon monoxide at the final follow up (after 12 months). 60 participants (13.8% of the total sample) were abstinent for 12 months. Of the 315 subjects, who had taken the drug, 49 (15.5%) stopped cytisine because of adverse effects (mostly gastric disturbances and nausea), although they were not serious. The long-term abstinence rates were similar to those observed in smokers receiving nicotine replacement therapy. Full-scale randomised trials of cytisine (Tabex), conducted to the standards required by regulatory authorities, were warranted.[122]

**Paul Aveyard et al (2008)-**A pragmatic randomised controlled trial was conducted to test the efficacy of nortriptyline plus nicotine replacement therapy compared with placebo plus nicotine replacement therapy for smoking cessation in 901 people trying to stop smoking at National Health Service stop smoking service clinics. Participants chose their nicotine replacement product, including combinations of nicotine replacement therapy,and received behavioural support. Nortriptyline was started one to two weeks before quit day, with the dose increased from 25mg to75mg daily for eight weeks and reduced if not tolerated. Primary outcome was prolonged confirmed abstinence at six months. Secondary outcomes were prolonged abstinence at 12 months, drug use, severity of side effects, nicotine withdrawal symptoms, and urge to smoke. 72 of 445 (16%) people using nortriptyline and 55 of 456 (12%) using placebo achieved prolonged abstinence at six months (relative risk 1.34, 95% confidence interval 0.97 to 1.86). At 12 months the corresponding values were 49 (11%) for nortriptyline and 40 (9%) for placebo (1.26, 0.84 to1.87). 337 (79%) people in the nortriptyline arm and 325 (75%) in the placebo arm were taking combination treatment on quit day, median 75 mg per day in both groups. More people in the nortriptyline arm than in the placebo arm took lower doses. The nortriptyline arm had noticeably higher severity ratings for dry mouth and constipation than the placebo arm, with slightly higher ratings for sweating and feeling shaky. Both groups had similar urges to smoke, but nortriptyline reduced depression and anxiety. Nortriptyline and nicotine replacement therapy are both effective for smoking cessation but the effect of the combination is less than either alone and evidence was lacking that combination treatment is more effective than either alone.[123]

**C. Neill Epperson et al (2010)-**A study examined the roles of gender, reproductive status and negative effect on smoking abstinence in subjects participating in a large (n=385) 6-week randomized clinical trial (RCT) of nicotine patch therapy, with varying doses of oral naltrexone (0 mg, 25 mg, 50 mg, 100 mg) treatment. Negative affect was assessed daily during the first post-quit week via telephone interactive voice response (IVR). Weight and adverse events were recorded weekly. In the intent to treat sample, the effects of dose on continuous abstinence were non-significant in the overall model for men and women. In the 295 study completers, there was a significant effect of dose on continuous abstinence in women only (F=8.53, $p$=0.04). In the 100 mg group, 71% of women were continuously abstinent compared to 41% in the placebo group ($p<0.05$).Women in the active naltrexone groups gained less weight (F=2.91, df=3, p=0.04). Women in the 100 mg versus placebo group were less adherent with medication (F=3.19, $p<0.05$). These effects were not significant in men. Naltrexone treatment condition (100 mg vs placebo, $p$=0.02, odds ratio (OR)= 0.28), gender (OR=0.55 $p$=0.09), and IVR ratings of negative affect (OR 1.02, *p*=0.04) predicted abstinence at Week-1 in study completers. Menstrual cycle status on quit day had a modest affect on abstinence. These data suggested that naltrexone dose, gender, and negative affect play a role in smoking abstinence, particularly in the early stages of treatment. When used in conjunction with nicotine replacement therapy, naltrexone dose might be important in women.[124]

**Gustavo Faibischew Prado et al (2011)-**A study was conducted to evaluate the effectiveness of nicotine replacement therapy (NRT), bupropion, nortriptyline and combination therapy and describe factors associated with treatment success. A total of 868 smokers (68.8% women) (meanage 49.6 years), the amount smoked was 25 cigarettes/day and the Fagerstrom Score was 6.6, attended a four-session cognitive-behavioural program and received medicines free of charge. Abstinence from smoking was assessed at each visit. Abstinence rates after 6 months and 1 year were 36.5% and 33.6%. In univariate analysis, male gender, age (.50), higher number of cigarettes smoked, cardiovascular comorbidities, longer interval from the last cigarette and combined treatment of nortriptyline plus NRT were predictive of abstinence, while neuropsychiatric comorbidities and the answer "yes" to the question "Do you smoke more often during the first hours after waking" were correlated with failure. In a multivariate model, predictors of abstinence were neuropsychiatric comorbidities, the answer "yes" to the question "Do you smoke more often during the first hours after waking" and combined treatment of nortriptyline plus NRT. Male gender and a longer period from the last cigarette were correlated with lower abstinence rate. Factors such as age, daily cigarette consumption, number of pack-years and dependency score were not reliable markers of abstinence. The combination nortriptyline+NRT was independently associated with higher abstinence rates.[125]

**Natalie Walker et al (2011)-**A single-blind, randomised controlled, non-inferiority trial designed to determine whether cytisine was at least as effective as NRT in assisting smokers to remain abstinent for at least one month. Participants (n = 1,310) recruited through the national telephone-based Quitline service in New Zealand and randomised to receive a standard 25-day course of cytosine tablets (Tabex®) or usual care (eight weeks of NRT patch and/or gum or lozenge). Participants in both study arms will also receive a behavioural support programme comprising an average of three follow-up telephone calls delivered over an eight-week period by Quitline. The primary outcome was continuous abstinence from smoking at one month, defined as not smoking more than five cigarettes since quit date. Outcome data collected at one week, two months and six months post-quit date. Cytisine appeared to be effective compared with placebo, and given its (current) relative low cost might be an acceptable smoking cessation treatment for smokers, particularly those in low-and middle-income countries. Cytisine's "natural" product status might also increase its acceptability and use among certain groups of smokers, such as indigenous people, smokers in countries where the use of natural medicines is widespread (e.g. China, India), and in those people who do not want to use NRT or anti-depressants to help them quit smoking. However it was important to ascertain the effectiveness of cytisine compared with that of existing cessation treatments.[126]

# DISCUSSION

Heavy tobacco use can lead to nicotine dependency. Nicotine's main acute effects over the cardiovascular system are peripheral vasoconstriction, increase of the blood pressure and heart rate. Nicotine also interferes with the endocrine system, yielding the release of antidiuretic hormone and water retention. In the gastrointestinal system, nicotine acts parasympathetically, stimulating tonus increase and intestinal motor activity. As CNS stimulant, leading to increased alertness, reduced appetite and sensations like dizziness, nausea and vomiting. Overall it affects individual's quality of life.

There are two types of interventions, namely non-pharmacological and pharmacological. Non-pharmacological interventions are important as they are cost effective such as Counselling by medical practitioners, Smoking cessation strategies delivered by nurses and support organizations, Telephonic call back and follow-up, health education and heavy taxation on tobacco products. When they are combined with pharmacological interventions, give better abstinence rates, even in resistant cases with frequent relapses. Various effective pharmacotherapeutic methods for tobacco cessation are now available and should be advised to the tobacco abusers. Pharmacotherapy should be strongly recommended to all persons with severe dependence, tobacco users with multiple failed self-attempts, tobacco users unable to abstain with brief intervention alone.

## NICOTINE REPLACEMENT THERAPY

Nicotine replacement therapies (NRTs) are smoking cessation medicines that contain nicotine, which is equally addictive, release small amounts of nicotine into the bloodstream to help counter cravings and reduce other physical withdrawal symptoms, enabling people to function better while dealing with the social and psychological aspects of their dependence. Nicotine replacement therapies increase the rate of long-term quitting by 50%–70%.[127]

Initially in 1990, researches experimented IV replacement of nicotine while cigarette smoking was permitted as desired, did not significantly affect the number of cigarettes smoked or amount of tobacco burnt, but nicotine intake from cigarettes was suppressed.[12]

**Analytes used for assessment:**

Knowledge of serum or urine concentration of analytes like Nicotine[14,15], trans-3 hydroxycotinine, nor nicotine[15] and anabasine[15,16] could be used to guide NRT or to assess tobacco abstinence in nicotine dependency treatment. These measurements have become an integral part of clinical treatment and management of patients who wish to overcome tobacco dependence.[15] Successful members of the NRT group made a significant greater reduction in their salivary cotinine scores.[17] Similarly, relationship between saliva and plasma cotinine concentration in a group of nicotine-dependent adolescent smokers could be a biomarker for abstinence but future research should seek to further validate saliva-to-plasma cotinine concentration ratios in adolescents.[18] Evaluating the behavioural impacton adherence of prescribing medication using genetic (DNA analysis) rather than phenotypic information could be an effective way. Adherence to NRT was greater among smokers informed that their oral dose of NRT is tailored to an analysis of DNA (genotype), compared to one tailored to nicotine dependence questionnaire score (phenotype).[19]

**Racial and ethnic variation**

Racial/ethnic variations in the use of nicotine replacement therapy (NRT) and quit ratios among Caucasian, African American, Asian, and Latino lifetime smokers were examined and it was found that Asian and Latino smokers were as likely as Caucasians to report smoking cessation and utilization rate in African Americans.[20]

Among African-American, high school students adolescent sample, NRT gum was used more often than the patch. But usually adolescent males, risk takers, and/or smokers appear more likely to use NRT (gum and/or patch) compared to their counter parts, despite limited empirical support for effective use of these products as cessation aids among adolescents.[21]

**Behavioural counselling**

Implementation of a guideline based smoking cessation intervention by intake clinicians in primary care was associated with higher abstinence among smokers.[23] NRT given with brief counselling to hospital inpatients was an effective routine smoking cessation intervention.[24] Regular face to face contact and monitoring of progress were particularly useful in helping to stop smoking, it provides compelling support for active promotion and support of smoking cessation.[22]A nurse managed smoking cessation intervention which included NRT also, could significantly increase cessation rates for hospitalized patients.[26] But NRT use by smokers making self initiated quit attempts without formal behavioural support would be associated with improved long-term abstinence rates.[25]

A Moore D, Aveyard Pet al concluded in his systematic review that replacement therapy was an effective intervention in achieving sustained smoking abstinence for smokers who have no intention or are unable to attempt an abrupt quit but it was unclear whether using nicotine replacement therapy without regular contact would be as effective.[128]

In a study in US, author found smoking counseling and NRT by physician increased from 16% of smoker's visit in 1991 to 29% in 1993 and decrease to 21% in 1995. They also suggested that a proportion of physicians were more likely to treat patients with smoking related diagnosis.[59]

**Telephone counseling**

Callers to the Minnesota QUITPLAN[SM] Helpline before and after the addition of access to free NRT was observed to assess change in cessation rates and programme impact, and author suggested increase in participation and abstinence rates resulting in an eight fold increase in programme impact.[28,29] Other studies also suggested that offering free NRT through a state quitline was an effective means of increasing quitline utilization and improving quit rates.[30,31,32,34] Whereas in another study author noted that telephone counselling by a nurse were ineffective in increasing quit rates. This form of assistance may be useful in the absence of physician advice, or when self selected by patients.[27]

Disadvantaged smokers were easily engaged to call the quitline, particularly when offered subsidized NRT. Disadvantaged smokers using the quitline, with and without subsidized NRT, achieved cessation outcomes comparable to other studies of "mainstream" smokers.[33]

**Over the counter availability and sale**

In 1996, US administration approved nicotine medication for OTC sale, which increased the use of medication by 152% compared with prior prescription use. Broader availability and promotion of effective treatments for tobacco dependence, specifically gums and patches increase the number of smokers availing themselves of the medications.[35] Other author also suggested OTC availability would result in more successful quitters, fewer smoking – attributable deaths and increased life expectancy for current smokers compared to prescription availability of NRT.[36,37]

Real-time monitoring of existing non traditional surveillance data, such as pharmacy sales of NRT products, could help assess the effects of public policies on cessation attempts. Increases in NRT product sales over the counter were observed during the weeks of the cigarette tax increases and the smoke-free workplace law in New York City, particularly in low-income areas.[39]

The Office of National Statistics (ONS) omnibus surveys showed no increase in the proportions of smokers making quit attempts and so the effects were solely on the proportions of quit attempts that were aided by medication. In the UK, making smoking cessation medicines reimbursable led to a large increase in utilization.[38]

Use of NRT increased short-term cessation success in moderate to heavy smokers whereas NRT appeared no longer effective in increasing long-term successful cessation in California smokers after becoming available over the counter.[40] Persistent uses of nicotine gum and patches were very rare and had not increased with the transition to OTC use, despite removal of physician oversight. [41]

In a study, no increase in smoker's rates of using NRT, making a quit attempt or stopping smoking was observed after NRT became available OTC sale. But there appeared to be other barriers to the use of NRT besides visiting a physician, especially among minority smokers.[42] In another study author described inappropriate use in adolescent smokers and non smokers for whom NRT is easily accessible and is used for reasons other than trying to quit smoking. Efforts are needed to discourage NRT use in non smokers' youth and to encourage appropriate use of NRT in young smokers to maximize its potential for successful cessation.[43]

Nicotine replacement products (nicotine gums and nicotine patches) play a significant role inreducing cigarette consumption, in addition to the negative effect of increasing cigarette price and the overall trend of declining cigarette consumption (as reflected by the time trend variable). This study suggested that additional efforts for promoting sales of nicotine replacement products will be another effective alternative to discouraging cigarette consumption.[44]

**Effectiveness**

NRT for aiding smoking reduction appeared to be safe. It was associated with a clinically significant reduction in smoke over a 5- week follow up and increase motivation to stop smoking.[45]

Mail survey of US smokers, NRT users (both ever-users and OTC users) were more likely to be older, male, and better educated. They were also heavier smokers, had experienced more craving and withdrawal upon quitting, and scored higher on measures of dependence.[46]

Smokers using pre-quitting NRT over two weeks appeared to titrate nicotine levels and symptoms of toxicity were uncommon and of low intensity.[50]

The sum of baseline days of NRT use and use of NRT on Day1 also predicted the"sum of days abstinent." Given NRT's effectiveness, but under utilization in real-world settings, the data support the need for interventions or strategies encouraging people to use NRT intheir quit attempts.[49]

In provision of providing free NRT, there were differences in the levels of interest: smokers who intended to quit were more interested in using the nicotine replacement therapy than those who planned to reduce or maintain their smoking.[47,48]

**Effect of NRT on Profile of Mood States (POMS)**

The effects of Nicotine Replacement Therapy (NRT) on the Profile of Mood States (POMS), testing whether pre-cessation depressive symptoms modify NRT's effects on POMS was evaluated and author suggested that those depressed in NRT conditions did not have significantly higher symptom scores compared to the non-depressed groups. In treating those negative moods NRT might be particularly important for persons with depressive symptoms before cessation.[51]

**NRT and systemic conditions**

Eliasson B et al said that the use of NRT during smoking cessation should be transient and limited because long term use of nicotine containing chewing gum was associated with insulin résistance and hyperinsulinemia[129] but the use of NRT is not associated with any increase in the risk of myocardial infarction, stroke, or death.[60]

In schizophrenic patients, pharmacotherapy strategies of higher dose nicotine patch, combining gum and patch, and augmentation medication to nicotine replacement should be evaluated in future.[52]

Pullon S et alwas conducted a postal survey among general practitioners and midwives about smoking cessation practice, and use of nicotine replacement therapy (NRT) during pregnancy and breastfeeding; respondents were uncertain about the safety of NRT use in pregnant and breastfeeding women and most of them requested more information about NRT use.[130]

It was feasible to recruit women for a trial of NRT in pregnancy as they wait for antenatal ultrasound examinations but women generally under-reported the amount they smoked on questionnaires completed whilst waiting in ultrasound department areas.[55]

In a study, it was found that infants exposed to NRT prenatally had an increased risk for infantile colic of the same magnitude as those exposed to tobacco smoke. Thus, nicotine might play a role in the pathogenesis of infantile colic.[56]

Adding a nicotine patch (15 mg per 16 hours) to behavioral cessation support for women who smoked during pregnancy did not significantly increase the rate of abstinence from smoking until delivery or the risk of adverse pregnancy or birth outcomes.[57]

Nicotine replacement therapy use was inconsistent following an initial quit attempt among methadone-maintained smokers. On days when NRT was used, individuals were likely to smoke at reduced levels or not at all.[54]

**Public Health Aspects**

Shiffman S et al found in a study that subjects who saw the advertisements framed as non commercial public announcement either a branded rather than as a promotion for or unbranded NRT products, were more likely to move away from cigarettes.[131]

West R et al suggested that the use of NRT for reasons other than quitting smoking may be more common than was previously estimated.A population based survey was done but did not find strong evidence that NRT use for purposes other than quitting smoking was either harmful or helpful.[132]

The potential impact of increased nicotine replacement therapy (NRT) use for smoking cessation was examined by comparing benefit and risk. Even after assuming some harm from long-term NRT use, the benefits from increased cessation success far outweigh the risks.[62]

Among different strategies to support smoking cessation i.e. no therapy, nicotine replacement (NRT), professional therapy and snus (snuff) use, Snuff was used commonly among men as a support for smoking cessation in Sweden. Women used pharmacological NRT to a greater extent, but this could probably not compensate for the much higher extent of snuff use as a cessation strategy among men.[58]

The low proportion of smokers being prescribed pharmacotherapeutic products strongly suggested that a major public health opportunity to prevent smoking related illness is being missed.[60]
In a comparison of the cost- effectiveness of a free nicotine replacement therapy (NRT) program with a statewide smoke-free workplace policy in Minnesota, Smoke-free workplace policies are about 9 times more cost-effective per new nonsmoker than free NRT programs are.[61]

The feasibility of engaging parents in a smoking cessation intervention at the time of a child's clinic visit might be an effective way to reach smokers who otherwise are unlikely to access smoking cessation interventions.[63]

Nicotine replacement therapy (NRT) when combined with counselling in young smokers in a deprived area of Nottingham, UK was unlikely to be effective in young smokers and also suggested that young smokers wanted help with smoking cessation, but establishing the efficacy of smoking cessation services for young people who need them most, would be very difficult.[64]

**Tobacco Cessation Centers**

First evaluation of a clinic-based smoking cessation service including NRT, in Asia showed that the service was acceptable to Chinese smokers.The quit rate in this pilot part-time clinic was comparable to those of full-time and better funded clinics in the West. A part-time smoking cessation clinic was a promising model for piloting smoking cessation services in the East.[65]

In the beginning 2002, a network of 19 tobacco cessation clinics (TCCs) was set up over a period of time to studythe feasibility of establishing tobacco cessation services in India. It was concluded that it is feasible to set up effective tobacco cessation clinics in developing countries.[66]

**VARIOUS NICOTINE REPLACEMENT THERAPY PRODUCTS**

**1. SILVER ACETATE**

Silver acetate chewing gum may be an alternative to nicotine-containing chewing gum when individuals have failed with the former product or when it is contraindicated. It demonstrated a modest benefit over placebo as a smoking deterrent in a minimal intervention and highly cost-effective treatment setting.[67]

A comparative study found no advantage from treatment with silver acetate chewing gum and only a short term advantage from treatment with nicotine chewing gum than ordinary chewing gum.[68]

**2. NICOTINE GUMS**

The usefulness of 2 mg nicotine chewing-gum as an aid to stop smoking was effective and implies a definite role for nicotine in cigarette dependence and withdrawal. Successful use of the gum requires careful attention to subjects' expectations and clear instructions on how to use it. Minor side effects were common but only gastric symptoms were more frequent with the active gum.[69]

A clear increase in the success rate was seen when the advice of general practitioners to stop smoking is accompanied by an offer of treatment with nicotine chewing gum. Author recommended that it would be feasible and effective for general practitioners to include the offer of nicotine gum and brief instructions on its use as part of a minimal intervention routine with all cigarette smokers.[70] Similarly, instructions and advice given by pharmacists might improve the smoking cessation rate in smokers receiving nicotine replacement therapy.[75]

Nicotine chewing gum is effective in improving the success rates in smoking cessation based on group therapy.[72] But in contrast, another author reported that the value of nicotine chewing gum, if any, can be quite small when it is used in general practice.[71]

The acute thermogenic effects of chewing gum containing different doses of nicotine and caffeine was assessed. Caffeine might be useful in preventing weight gain after smoking cessation if its thermogenic effect can be used to enhance nicotin's effect on long-term energy balance. [74]

Combination of sublingual pralidoxime and ipratropium (ProBAN) together combined with nicotine gum doubled the continuous sustained quit rate compared with nicotine replacement alone, with no adverse effects. Although not statistically significant due to the size of the study, this result suggests that it may be an effective therapy for smoking cessation, and larger studies are warranted.[73]

In an estimation of the safety and efficacy of treatment with 2 mg nicotine gum for smoking cessation in pregnant women who smoked daily, received individualized behavioural counselling, author suggested that despite not reducing smoking during pregnancy, use of nicotine gum increased birth weight and gestational age, two key parameters in predicting neonatal wellbeing.[76]

## 3. TRANSDERAML PATCHES

All transdermal nicotine doses significantly decreased the severity of nicotine withdrawal symptoms and significantly reduced cigarette use by patients who did not stop smoking. Compliance was excellent, and no serious systemic adverse effects were reported. Transdermal nicotine systems showed considerable promise as an aid to smoking cessation.[77,84] Patches were most effective for smokers with moderate nicotine dependence and for younger smokers specially.[80]

The use of 42 mg/day nicotine patch therapy is safe and should be considered initial therapy in the clinical setting among Smokeless Tobacco users who use $\geq$ 3 cans per week.[86]

Randomized trial on transdermal patch showed that Genetically, DRD2 genetic variants, related to relatively decreased dopaminergic tone in the mesocorticolimbic system were associated with increased risk for relapse to smoking following a cessation attempt.[87] Genetic variation in the dopamine pathway might provide a future basis for tailored smoking cessation therapies, but indicated that different genes influencing various components of this pathway might have different effects on response to smoking cessation pharmacotherapy.[89]

Transdermal nicotine patches used as an adjunct to brief advice and support in a general practice setting are an effective aid to long term cessation of smoking in highly dependent smokers.[79] Also, when it was used as an adjunct to low-intervention therapy, significantly reduced tobacco withdrawal symptoms and enhanced smoking cessation rates.[78] Similarly, Contingent vouchers (participants received vouchers contingent on abstinence from smoking), were more effective than transdermal nicotine patches in promoting abstinence.[88]

High-dose transdermal nicotine has the potential to substantially suppress the intake of tobacco smoke and could be a useful strategy for smoking cessation therapy or for reducing the harm caused by smoking[83,85] and it may delay post cessation weight gain for both men and women but factors that predict weight change with long-term abstinence from smoking could not be identified.[81]

Nicotine patch use in smokers who purchased the product as a non-prescription medicine from pharmacies was assessed and preliminary data on the non-prescription usage of transdermal nicotine when purchased through pharmacies was recorded. Twenty-eight per cent of respondents reported continuing smoking, although the number of cigarettes smoked was much less, than in the reported smoking history. Side effects were reported by 24% of patch users, but there was no evidence of significant safety problems.[82]

The feasibility of formulating mucoadhesive buccal nicotine patches, prepared using xanthan gum or carbopol as a mucoadhesive polymers and ethyl cellulose as a backing layer was observed in an invitro study. Author suggested that xanthan patches showed a reasonable fast initial release profile followed by controlled drug release over a 10-h period.[90]

## 4. NICOTINE GUMS AND PATCHES

Among the most highly nicotine dependent smokers the 4 mg gum is the most effective form of replacement therapy and in less highly dependent smokers the different preparations are comparable in their efficacy but the patch offers greater convenience and minimal need for instruction in its use.[91]

Smokers without alcohol problems showed that combination therapy (nicotine patch plus gum) was more effective than monotherapy (nicotine patch) for smoking cessation.[92]

## 5. NASAL NICOTINE INHALAR:

The more rapid and efficient absorption of nicotine from the nasal nicotine solution than from nicotine chewing gum suggests that it might prove a useful aid to giving up smoking. It might be particularly useful in smokers for whom the gum is less suitable on account of dentures or peptic ulcers or who experience nausea and dyspeptic symptoms from the gum.[93]Another author also suggested that Nicotine inhaler appeared safe to use and increased success rates of smoking cessation attempts. The treatment was well tolerated, and no serious adverse events were reported.[94]

In an evaluation of the efficacy and safety of nicotine 4 mg gum or nicotine 10 mg inhaler in helping smokers to reduce or quit smoking, both resulted in a significantly higher abstinence rate than placebo. In addition a large number of smokers managed to reduce their cigarette consumption by more than 50% compared to baseline.[98]

Similarly, the efficacy of the nicotine inhaler plus nicotine patch vs nicotine inhaler plus placebo patch for smoking cessation was compared, author reported that treatment with the nicotine inhaler plus nicotine patch resulted in significantly higher cessation rates than inhaler plus placebo patch[96] whereas in other study, author found that in hospital patients, NRT given as regular daily patches plus an inhalator to be used as needed, did not add to the smoking cessation rate achieved at 1 year by regular advice and support, despite significantly increasing the cessation rate at 1 week.[97]

In a comparison to monitor the effect of a novel nicotine delivery device (Eclipse) on cigarette smoking, carbon monoxide and nicotine concentrations, and motivation to give up smoking with the smoker's own brand of cigarette and Nicotrol inhaler. Eclipse can dramatically decrease cigarette consumption without causing withdrawal symptoms or decreases in nicotine concentrations or motivation to quit altogether. Unlike the inhaler, Eclipse produces an increase in carbon monoxide concentration so it may not be a safer cigarette.[95]

### 6. NICOTINE SPRAY:

A trial, to assess the impact of instructional guidance in the regular use of use nicotine nasal spray (NNS) on the true use of NNS, recommended the use of NNS only when craving appeared for heavy smokers willing to quit seems acceptable compared to prescribing hourly administration. [101]

In a comparison among nicotine polacrilex (gum), a transdermal patch, nasal spray, and an inhaler, the products did not differ in their effects on withdrawal discomfort, urges to smoke, or rates of abstinence. Compliance with recommended nicotine replacement treatment use was high for the patch, low for gum, and very low for the spray and the inhaler. The spray was under used because of adverse effects more often than the other products. [99] Another study also suggested that the unpleasant side effects like nasal irritation and burning followed by complaints about the taste and smell, poor adherence, and consequent lack of efficacy observed in randomized open label trial did not support the use of nicotine nasal spray as an adjunct to counseling for adolescent smokers wishing to quit. [100]

## 7. NICOTINE LOZENGES:

A study tested the safety and efficacy of nicotine polacrilex (2- and 4-mg nicotine lozenges) for smoking cessation. Smokers who used more lozenges achieved significantly better treatment effects. Use of the active lozenge also resulted in reduced craving and withdrawal. Most adverse events were moderate and resembled those seen with nicotine gum. The nicotine lozenge was a safe and effective new treatment for smoking cessation in low- and high-dependence smokers.[102]Another study determined if the 4-mg nicotine lozenge with a behavioural intervention could facilitate smokeless tobacco (ST) use reduction among ST users compared with a behavioural intervention alone, author found the use of reduction strategies for ST users not interested in quitting deserves further evaluation as an intervention strategy. [103]

In contrast, a randomized trial compared the effectiveness of transdermal nicotine vs. nicotine lozenge for smoking cessation, the author found Transdermal nicotine may be more effective than nicotine lozenge for smokers who prefer transdermal nicotine and do not smoke to alleviate emotional distress or stimulate cognitive function.[104]

## NON NICOTINE REPLACEMENT THERAPY PRODUCTS

In this type of the therapy, medication which acts on central brain receptors on similar set of neurotransmitters that are affected by nicotine and minimize withdrawal from nicotine when the tobacco user suddenly stops use.

The context in which phamacotheraputic agents both NRT and bupropion are prescribed in UK general practice and whether guidelines are being followed were examined, author recommended that more active implementation of guidelines could increase the impact of general practice on the prevalence of smoking. [105]

GPs vary in their beliefs about the effectiveness and safety of smoking cessation medications. Their intentions to prescribe these medications vary in line with beliefs as about effectiveness of NRT and bupropion and the perceived danger of bupropion and about neglecting psychological aspects of smoking and incorrect use had indirect effects on intentions to prescribe NRT without support. Interventions aimed at increasing the likelihood with which GPs prescribe these medications might be more effective if they addressed these beliefs. [106]

**BUPROPION**

Bupropion works by blocking the dopamine transporter pump preventing the transport of dopamine back into the neuron, and thereby increasing the amount of dopamine in the synaptic cleft. It is therefore classified as an antidepressant.

In adouble-blind study for placebo and a sustained-release form of bupropion for smoking cessation, the rates of smoking cessation was significantly better than those for the placebo group. Author concluded a sustained-release form of bupropion was effective for smoking cessation and was accompanied by reduced weight gain and minimal side effects. [107] Another study also evaluated sustained released Bupropion as an effective aid for smoking cessation which was well tolerated by the respondents. The most commonly reported adverse effects were insomnia, headache and dry mouth.[117]

In a comparison of sustained release bupropion, a nicotine patch, bupropion and a nicotine patch, and placebo for smoking cessation, abstinence rates were higher with combination therapy than with bupropion alone, but the difference was not statistically significant. [108] Whereas another study suggested that there was a trend toward increased quit rates among participants randomized to bupropion in comparison with placebo group but author also suggested that, 7-week bupropion trial to treatment with nicotine replacement therapy and counselling did not significantly increase smoking cessation rates.[111]

In a population-based clinical trial, smokers in primary care practices had been offered them a free treatment course of either bupropion or transdermal nicotine replacement (TNR). Of the smokers requesting pharmacotherapy, 51% requested bupropion and 49% requested TNR. Choice of bupropion was related to no history of heart disease and no previous use of bupropion. [114]

In a study for assessing cost effectiveness of three smoking cessation strategies based on pharmacotherapies, the cost-effectiveness ratios for both nicotine gums and patches were higher than that for bupropion. Author concluded that Bupropion treatment for 1 year would prevent a greater number of deaths than the alternative strategies due to the decrease in the number of smokers. When assessing interventions and their costs economic evaluation shows that in the long run greater use of bupropion generates net savings in tobacco-related health costs.[110] Another author also agreed to cost effectiveness property of Bupropion in comparison with NRT (nicotine patches and nicotine gums) in smoking cessation programs that has been followed for 20 years. Author found that the incremental costs per QALY (quality-adjusted life-year) gained were relatively low for bupropion in comparison to nicotine patches in Swedish kronas and concluded Bupropion is a cost-effective therapy in smoking cessation programs. [112]

Whereas Bertram MY et al concluded that, compared with other drugs, bupropion and NRT are both highly cost-effective in smoking cessation interventions. [113] Study showed nicotine replacement therapy (NRT) and bupropion were generally perceived as effective and cost-effective. But GPs perceived bupropion as dangerous and were concerned about its side effects. [106]

A laboratory study examined the effects of 300 mg/day bupropion, compared with placebo. Significant interactions indicated that bupropion reduced the effects of acute abstinence on smoking urges in the presence of neutral cues, only in those who intended to quit.[115] A study was done to directly compare of the short-term validated abstinence rates of NRT and bupropion in a clinical setting. Abstinence rate in clients using NRT was higher than for bupropion because Obtaining NRT was relatively easy for clients throughout the study period whilst this was not the case for bupropion. So it was suggested that implementation issues and/or self-selection might influence the effectiveness of medications in health care, as opposed to research, settings.[109]

## 2. VARENICLINE

In a comparision of 12-week standard regimen of varenicline with a 10-week standard regimen of transdermal nicotine replacement therapy (NRT) for smoking cessation, Varenicline significantly reduced craving ($p < 0.001$), withdrawal symptoms ($p < 0.001$)and smoking satisfaction ($p < 0.001$) compared with NRT.[118]

A study analysed the cost effectiveness of varenicline compared with bupropion, NRT (nicotine replacement therapy) and no pharmacological treatment in Spain. Author concluded that varenicline was cost-effective in comparison with any other alternative. Varenicline was a dominant option (more effective at a lower cost) compared with all other smoking cessation treatments when the time frame is the life span of the patient.[119]

Varenicline had statistically significant increased risk of reported depression and suicidal/selfinjurious behavior as compared to Bupropion. The findings for varenicline, combined with other problems with its safety profile, render it unsuitable for first-line use in smoking cessation.[120]

## 3. OTHERS

In 21-mg nicotine patch and oral naltrexone hydrochloride clinical trial after equal random treatment assignment, the 100-mg dose of naltrexone hydrochloride appears the most promising for augmenting the efficacy of the nicotine patch on smoking cessation outcomes. The significant weight reduction with low-dose naltrexone therapy suggested that it might be useful as a second-line treatment for weight concerned smokers.[121]

A study examined the roles of gender, reproductive status and negative effect on smoking abstinence with nicotine patch therapy and varying doses of oral naltrexone. The data suggested that naltrexone dose, gender, and negative affect play a role in smoking abstinence, particularly in the early stages of treatment. When used in conjunction with nicotine replacement therapy, naltrexone dose might be important in women.[124]

The long-term abstinence rates were similar for cytisine (Tabex) to those observed in smokers receiving nicotine replacement therapy. Adverse effects (mostly gastric disturbances and nausea) were not serious.[122] Cytisine's "natural" product status might increase its acceptability and use among certain groups of smokers, such as indigenous people, smokers in countries where the use of natural medicines is widespread (e.g. China, India), and in those people who do not want to use NRT or anti-depressants to help them quit smoking. [126]

In a randomised controlled trial to test the efficacy of nortriptyline plus nicotine replacement therapy compared with placebo, author suggested that, both groups had similar urges to smoke, but nortriptyline reduced depression and anxiety. Nortriptyline and nicotine replacement therapy are both effective for smoking cessation but the effect of the combination is less than either alone and evidence was lacking that combination treatment is more effective than either alone.[123] whereas another study evaluated the effectiveness of nicotine replacement therapy (NRT), bupropion, nortriptyline and combination therapy. Abstinence from smoking was assessed at each visit. The combination nortriptyline+NRT was independently associated with higher abstinence rates.[125]

Hence, Pharmacotherapy has valuable role in treating tobacco dependence. Tobacco dependence is a chronic, relapsing medical illness. In India, it is estimated that nearly one million deaths occur due to tobacco use every year. There are two main interventions to facilitate tobacco user cessation. The first is counseling, including face-to-face advice from physicians and other health-care workers incorporated into regular medical care as well as over the telephone via quit lines and community programmes. The other is pharmacological therapy. Advantages of pharmacotherapy include increase in quit rates and in helping the person to effectively make life changes to quit tobacco and its disadvantages include limited availability, cost and side-effects. All forms of NRT (gum, patches and inhaler), bupropion and varenicline are safe and effective for increasing smoking cessation rates in the short and long terms. The effectiveness of drug treatments is multiplied when associated with effective counseling or behavioural treatments. Choice of medication depends primarily on adverse effects, medical contraindications, psychiatric morbidity, concurrent medication, cost, patient preference.

NRT and other pharmacological treatments for nicotine addiction are comparatively safe if used as directed, and they are unlikely to cause adverse behavioural, cardiovascular, or other health effects. NRT can be prescribed to persons with underlying stable cardiovascular disease, including angina and previous myocardial infarction. NRTs may be prescribed to pregnant and lactating mothers to help them quit under medical supervision. NRTs are not solutions in themselves to the public health problem of cigarette use. Rather, their use must be considered as part of comprehensive prevention and cessation programs.

Since 2001, the Ministry of Health and Family Welfare (MoH&FW) has, with support from WHO, established 19 tobacco cessation centres in 17 states across the country in diverse settings such as cancer treatment hospitals, psychiatric hospitals, medical colleges and NGOs to help users quit the tobacco addiction. The 2007 five-year National Tobacco Control Programme proposed to set up additional cessation centres in 450 districts. Services are provided through various tools such as behavioural counselling, pharmacotherapy and a combination therapy after assessing the degree of nicotine dependence of the tobacco user. But regarding pharmacotherapy, only Nicotine gums and lozenges are available over the counter and in most of the states less than 2 percent of smokers used pharmacotherapy for cessation. The high prevalence of tobacco use in India calls for urgent action. Only a concerted effort could realize a dream of tobacco free world.

# CONCLUSION

Ironically, after five centuries, tobacco has gone from a medicinal plant to one of the worst world public health issues. Nicotine is the primary component of tobacco. It is recognized as one of the most frequently used addictive drugs, and it is very important for tobacco users to quit.

Counselling is an effective and cost-effective method for smoking cessation, but counselling alone may not be useful for chronic smokers and its effectiveness can be improved by simultaneous pharmacotherapy.

Pharmacological intervention leads to a near doubling of cessation rates achieved by non-pharmacological intervention, irrespective of the level of that intervention. It will therefore increase the chance of success with any quit attempt but ismost effective when combined with intensive behavioural support.

Several randomized, double-blind, placebo- controlled trials related to pharmacotherapy, have reported significantly higher abstinence rates with first-line, and some second-line, drugs compared with placebo. These clinical trials provide scientific evidence of the efficacy and safety of nicotine replacement therapy (NRT), bupropion , varenicline as first line drugs and clonidine and nortriptyline used as second-line smoking cessation therapy; however, the effectiveness and limitations of these drug regimens in real-life settings are still poorly documented.

NRT has become the standard of care for the treatment of tobacco dependence to facilitate smoking cessation. It is the most widely used pharmacological adjunct to advice and behavioural support when treating tobacco dependence. Because it is safe for virtually all smokers and is the only medicine easily available over the counter and on general sale, it is likely to remain the most popular treatment for the foreseeable future. NRT partially replaces the nicotine from cigarettes over the initial 8–12 week period of stopping smoking. It reduces tobacco withdrawal symptoms during the period when they are most severe, enabling the smoker time to adjust to life without cigarettes. The choice of the NRT to be used depends on comorbid conditions, previous use and the need for rapid delivery of NRT. In highly dependent patients, measures delivering a higher dose of nicotine, such as a nasal spray or an inhaler, would be preferred.

Bupropion is effective in nicotine-dependency treatment; however there are several clinical conditions that contraindicate its use. Nicotine replacement therapy presents good outcomes when associated with bupropion, although it also has limitations, besides not being considered for patients with severe cardiovascular diseases. It is seen that bupropion may be more effective as an anti smoking treatment in people who are motivated to quit because low doses of bupropion produce a nicotine-like effect that serves as a suitable substitute.

Varenicline was developed significantly for smoking cessation and it demonstrated both short and long term efficacy. It doubles or triples the chances of quitting. It has been reported to be well tolerated and appears to attenuate the urge to smoke.

Both NRT and non NRT are effective and established pharmacotherapies for smoking cessation, but require an office visit to get a prescription and are generally more costly compared to several formulations of NRT available over the counter.

The most important aim of any intervention for smoking cessation should be the prevention of a relapse after successful therapy. A return to smoking after 1-2 weeks of abstinence is very common, which is more so in previously depressed patients or patients dependent on alcohol. Bupropion is effective in such patients and it also effectively abolishes nicotine withdrawal symptoms.

It is also difficult to evaluate the efficacy of NRT and bupropion when self-administered. It is predicted that though they increase the initial quit rate, in the long-term, there is poor compliance and early discontinuation.

However, the role of willingness to quit cannot be undermined. Despite the broad therapeutic armamentarium available, smoking cessation is still a therapeutic challenge all around the world.

# FUTURESCOPE

1. **RIMONABANT (SR 141716)-** Rimonabant is a selective cannabinoid receptor antagonist which blocks the CB-1 receptor. In animal studies, it has shown beneficial effects in treating obesity, smoking cessation and metabolic syndrome. In human studies, rimonabant has been effective in the treatment of obesity and smoking cessation. To date only nausea is reported to be greater than placebo. Animal studies suggested suggesting that it is not only effective in smoking cessation, but also capable of maintaining abstinence.

2. **NICOTINE VACCINE** Currently under Phase II trials, the nicotine vaccine acts by inducing nicotine specific antibodies which can combine with nicotine in the blood and prevent nicotine's entry into the brain, thereby reducing its addictive potential and preventing a relapse following smoking cessation.

3. **TOPIRAMATE-** It is an AMPA/kainite antagonist and thus could be of value in the treatment of addiction. A small study, comprising 13 subjects, has shown this agent of some value in the pharmacotherapy of smoking cessation.

4. **GLUCOSE TABS -** Single doses of nicotine relieve hunger in smokers and hunger pangs, sometimes, are associated with a craving for cigarettes. The adaptation to long-term nicotine intake leads to the exacerbation of these sensations during periods of abstinence. The low cost of glucose tablets can make it a useful adjunct in smoking cessation treatment.

5. **MECAMYLAMINE-** It is a nicotine antagonist and mayblock the rewarding effect of nicotine, thereby reducing the urge to smoke. The combination of mecamylamine with nicotine and the placebo showed a highest abstinence rate of 40% and statistically significant benefit with mecamylamine.

6. **D $_3$ RECEPTOR LIGANDS** -Pharmacological and behavioural evidence implicates dopamine D $_3$ receptors in the mechanisms underlying stimulus controlled drug seeking behaviour. D $_3$ receptor ligands would be selective for rewarding and reinforcing the effects of nicotine which contribute to tobacco smoking behaviour, without affecting subjective responses to nicotine or producing any antidepressant-like effect.

7. **TRYPTOPHAN AND HIGH CARBOHYDRATE DIET** -Serotonin enhancing substances such as tryptophan and high carbohydrate diets have been shown to reduce the negative effect, which is also a classic symptom of withdrawal. Tryptophan and high carbohydrate diet could become an important adjuvant in smoking cessation therapy.

# REFERENCES


1. ReddyS.K., Gupta P.C. Report on Tobacco Control in India. Ministryof Health & Family Welfare, GOI. 2004.Pages 8-11.
2. Gauravi A. Mishra, Parishi V. Majmudar, Subhadra D. Gupta, Pallavi S. Rane, PallaviA.Uplap,SurendraS.Shastri.Workplacetobacco cessation program in India:A successstory.Indian J Occup Environ Med. 2009 Dec; 13(3): 146–153.
3. WHO (2008), MPOWER: a policy package to reverse the tobacco epidemic. Mpower: a policy package to reverse the tobacco epidemic. WHO Press, World Health Organization, Switzerland.
4. Gupta P.C. The public health impact of tobacco. Current Science.2001 Sep;81(5): 475-481.
5. Herrick C., Herrick C., Mitchell M. 100 Questions & Answers About How to Quit Smoking. 1st Edition USA: Jones and Bartlett Publishers; 2010.pages 92-117.
6. WHO (2017), Regional Office for Africa: Chapter1, Types of Tobacco Use.
7. Smokeless Tobacco: Health Effects, CDC; https://www.cdc.gov/tobacco/data_statistics/fact_sheets/smokeless/health_effects/index.htm
8. Health effects of Cigarette Smoking, CDC; https://www.cdc.gov/tobacco/data_statistics/fact_sheets/health_effects/effects_cig_smoking/index.htm
9. Tobacco dependence treatment guidelines. National Tobacco control programme. Directorate general of Health services, Ministry of family and health welfare. Government of India.2011: p.7-11.
10. Rabius V, Pike KJ, Hunter J, Wiatrek D, McAlister AL. Effects of frequency and duration in telephone counselling for smoking cessation. Tob Control. 2007Dec;16 Suppl 1(Suppl 1):i71-4.
11. Helping People Quit Tobacco: A Manual for Doctors and Dentists. World Health Organization, Regional Office for South-East Asia.2010:p. 85-96.
12. Benowitz NL, Zevin S, Jacob P.Intravenous nicotine replacement suppresses nicotine intake from cigarette smoking. JPET 1990; 254(3): 1000-1005.
13. Buck D, Morgan. A Smoking and quitting with the aid of Nicotine Replacement Therapies in the English adult population: Results from the Health Education Monitoring Survey 1995; Eur J Public Health2001; 11(2): 211-217.

14. Paoletti P, Fornai E, Maggiorelli F, Puntoni R, Viegi G, Carrozzi L, et al: Importance of baseline cotinine plasma values in smoking cessation: results from a double-blind study with nicotine patch. Eur Respir J 1996; 9: 643–651.

15. Moyer TP, Charlson JR, Enger RJ, Dale LC, Ebbert JO, Schroeder DR, Hurt RD. Simultaneous analysis of nicotine, nicotine metabolites and tobacco alkaloids in serum or urine bytandem mass spectrometry, with clinically relevant metabolic profiles. Clin Chem 2002; 48(9):1460-71.

16. Jacob P 3rd, Hatsukami D, Severson H, Hall S, Yu L, Benowitz NL. Anabasine and anatabine as biomarkers for tobacco use during nicotine replacement therapy; Cancer Epidemiol Biomarkers Prev. 2002 Dec; 11(12):1668-73.

17. Croucher R, Islam S, Jarvis MJ. Oral tobacco cessation with UK resident Bangladeshi women: a community pilot investigation; Health Educ Res. 2003 Apr; 18(2):216-23.

18. Parzynski CS, Jaszyna-Gasior M, Franken FH, Moolchan ET. Measuring nicotine intake among highly dependent adolescent smokers: comparability of saliva andplasma cotinine concentrations; Pharmacol Biochem Behav. 2008 Apr; 89(2):145-9.

19. Marteau TM, Munafò MR, Aveyard P, Hill C, Whitwell S, Willis TA, et al. Trial Protocol:Using genotype to tailor prescribing of nicotine replacement therapy: a randomized controlled trial assessing impact of communication upon adherence; BMC Public Health. 2010 Nov 9; 10: 680-689.

20. Fu SS, Kodl MM, Joseph AM, Hatsukami DK, Johnson EO, Breslau N, et al. Racial/Ethnic disparities in the use of nicotine replacement therapy and quit ratios in lifetime smokers ages 25 to 44 years; Cancer Epidemiol Biomarkers Prev.2008 Jul;17(7):1640-7.

21. Dalton WT 3rd, Klesges LM. Gender, smoking status, and risk behavior attitudes explain adolescents' patterns of nicotine replacement therapy use; Addict Behav. 2010 Feb; 35(2):147-51.

22. Cruse S.M., Forster N. J. D., Thurgood G.and Sys L. Smoking cessation in the workplace: results of an intervention programme using nicotine patches. Occup Med (Lond) 2001; 51 (8):501-506.

23. Katz DA, Muehlenbruch DR, Brown RL, Fiore MC, Baker TB. Effectiveness of implementing the agency for health care research and quality smoking

cessation clinical practice guideline: a randomized, controlled trial, J Natl Cancer Inst. 2004 Apr 21;96(8):594-603.

24. Molyneux A, Lewis S, Leivers U. Clinical trial comparing nicotine replacement therapy (NRT) plus brief counselling, brief counseling alone, and minimal intervention on smoking cessation in hospital inpatients. Thorax. 2003 Jun; 58(6):484-8.

25. Johnstone EC, Elliot KM, David SP, Murphy MF, Walton RT, Munafò MR. Association of COMTVal108/158 Met genotype with smoking cessation in a nicotine replacement therapy randomized trial; Cancer Epidemiol Biomarkers Prev. 2007 Jun;16(6):1065-9.

26. Taylor C B, Miller N H. A Nurse-Managed Smoking Cessation Program for Hospitalized Smokers. Am J Public Health 1996; 86(11):1557–1560.

27. Reid R D, Pipe A, Dafoe W A. Is telephone counselling a useful addition to physician advice and nicotine replacement therapy in helping patients to stop smoking? A randomized controlled trial. CMAJ 1999; 160:1577-81.

28. An LC, Schillo BA, Kavanaugh AM, Lachter RB, Luxenberg MG, Wendling AH, et al. Increased reach and effectiveness of a statewide tobacco quitline after the addition of access to free nicotine replacement therapy; Tob Control. 2006 Aug; 15(4):286-93.

29. Wilson N, Sertsou G, Edwards R, Thomson G, Grigg M, Li J. A new national smokefree law increased calls to a national quitline; BMC Public Health. 2007 May 8;7:75.

30. Schillo BA, Wendling A. Expanding access to nicotine replacement therapy through Minnesota's QUITLINE partnership; Tob Control. 2007 Dec; 16 Suppl 1:i37-41.

31. Tinkelman D, Wilson SM, Willett J, Sweeney CT. Offering free NRT through a tobacco quitline: impact on utilisation and quit rates; Tob Control. 2007 Dec; 16 Suppl 1:i42-6.

32. Hollis JF, McAfee TA, Fellows JL, Zbikowski SM, Stark M, Riedlinger K. The effectiveness and cost effectiveness of telephone counselling and the nicotine patch in a state tobacco quitline; Tob Control. 2007 Dec; 16 Suppl 1:i53-9.

33. Miller CL, Sedivy V. Using A quitline plus low cost nicotine replacement therapy to help disadvantaged smokers to quit; Tob Control. 2009 Apr; 18(2):144-9.

34. Saul JE, LienR, Schillo B, Kavanaugh A, Wendling A, Luxenberg M, et al. Outcomes and cost effectiveness of two nicotine replacement treatment delivery models for a tobacco quitline; Int J Environ Res Public Health.2011 May; 8(5):1547-59.

35. Shiffmen S, Gitchell J, Pinney M, Burton S L, Kemper K E, Lara E A, et al. Public health benefit of over the counter nicotine medications. Tobacco Control 1997; 6: 306-310.

36. Lawrence WF, Smith SS, Baker TB, Fiore MC. Does over-the-counter nicotine replacement therapy improve smokers' life expectancy? Tobacco Control 1998; 7:364–368.

37. Reed MB, Anderson CM, Vaughn JW, Burns DM. The effect of over-the-counter sales of the nicotine patch and nicotine gum on smoking cessation in California; Cancer Epidemiol Biomarkers Prev. 2005 Sep; 14(9):2131-6.

38. West R, Di Marino ME, Gitchell J, McNeill A. Impact of UK policy initiatives on use of medicines to aid smoking cessation; Tob Control. 2005 Jun; 14(3):166-71.

39. Metzger KB, Mostashari F, Kerker BD. Use of pharmacy data to evaluate smoking regulations' impact on sales of nicotine replacement therapies in New York City; Am J Public Health. 2005 Jun; 95(6):1050-5.

40. Pierce JP, Gilpin EA. Impact of over-the counter sales on effectivenessof pharmaceuticalaids for smoking cessation; JAMA. 2002 Sep 11; 288(10):1260-4.

41. Shiffman S, Hughes JR, Pillitteri JL, Burton SL. Persistent use of nicotine replacement therapy: an analysis of actual purchase patterns in a population based sample; Tob Control. 2003 Sep; 12(3):310-6.

42. Thorndike AN, Biener L, Rigotti NA.. Effect on smoking cessation of switching nicotine replacement therapy to over-the-counter status. Am J Public Health 2002; 92(3):437-42.

43. Klesges LM, Johnson KC, Somes G, Zbikowski S, Robinson L. Use of nicotine replacement therapy in adolescent smokers and nonsmokers; Arch Pediatr Adolesc Med. 2003 Jun;157(6):517-22.

44. Hu T, Sung HY, Keeler TE, Marciniak M. Cigarette consumption and sales of nicotine replacement products. Tobacco Control. 2000; 9 Suppl 2:1160-3.

45. Fagerstrom K.O., Tejding R, Westin A, Lunell E. Aiding reduction of smoking with nicotine replacement medications : hope for the recalcitrant smoker? Tobacco control 1997; 6: 311-316

46. Shiffman S, Di Marino ME, Sweeney CT. Characteristics of selectors of nicotine replacement therapy, Tob Control. 2005 Oct; 14(5):346-55.

47. Cunningham JA, Selby PL. Intentions of smokers to use free nicotine replacement therapy; CMAJ. 2008 Jul 15; 179(2):145-6.

48. Cunningham JA, Leatherdale ST, Selby PL, Tyndale RF, Zawertailo L, Kushnir V. Randomized controlled trial of mailed Nicotine
Replacement Therapy to Canadian smokers: study protocol; BMC Public Health. 2011 Sep 28; 11:741

49. Amodei N, Lamb RJ. The role of nicotine replacement therapy in early quitting success; Nicotine Tob Res. 2010 Jan; 12(1):1-10.

50. Chris Bullen, Robyn Whittaker, Natalie Walker, Mark Wallace-Bell. Pre-quitting nicotine replacement therapy: Findings from a pilot study; Tobacco Induced Diseases. 2006; 3(2):35-40.

51. Korhonen T, Kinnunen TH, Garvey AJ. Impact of Nicotine Replacement Therapy on post-cessation mood profile by pre-cessation depressive symptoms; Tob Induc Dis. 2006 Aug 15;3(2):17-33.

52. Ziedonis DM, George TP. Schizophrenia and Nicotine Use: Report of a Pilot Smoking Cessation Program and Review of Neurobiological and Clinical Issues. Schizophrenia Bulletin 1997; 23(2): 247-254.

53. Hubbard R, Lewis S, Smith C, Godfrey C, Smeeth L, Farrington P, et al. Use of nicotine replacement therapy and the risk of acute myocardial infarction, stroke, and death; Tob Control. 2005 Dec;14(6):416-21

54. Stein MD, Anderson BJ, Niaura R. Nicotine replacement therapy: patterns of use after a quit attempt among methadone-maintained smokers; J Gen Intern Med. 2006 Jul; 21(7):753-7.

55. Coleman T, Antoniak M, Britton J, Thornton J, Lewis S, Watts K. Recruiting pregnant smokers for a placebo-randomised controlled trial of nicotine replacement therapy; BMC Health Serv Res. 2004 Nov 1;4(1):29.

56. Milidou I, Henriksen TB, Jensen MS, Olsen J, Søndergaard C. Nicotine replacement therapy during pregnancy and infantile colic in the offspring; Pediatrics. 2012 Mar; 129(3):e652-8.

57. Coleman T, Cooper S, Thornton JG, Grainge MJ, Watts K, Britton J, et al. A Randomized Trial of Nicotine- Replacement Therapy Patches in Pregnancy, N Engl J Med 2012; 366:808-818.

58. Lindström M. Nicotine replacement therapy, professional therapy, snuff use and tobacco smoking: a study of smoking cessation strategies in southern Sweden; Tob Control. 2007 Dec; 16(6):410-6.

59. Thorndike AN, Rigotti NA, Stafford RS, Singer DE. National Patterns in the Treatment of Smokers by Physicians. JAMA 1998; 279:604-608.

60. Wilson A, Hippisley-Cox J, Coupland C, Coleman T, Britton J, Barrett S. Smoking cessation treatment in primary care: prospective cohort study, Tob Control. 2005 Aug; 14(4):242-6.

61. Ong MK, Glantz SA. Free nicotine replacement therapy programs vs implementing smoke-free workplaces: a cost-effectiveness comparison; Am J Public Health.2005 Jun; 95(6):969-75.

62. Apelberg BJ, Onicescu G, Avila-Tang E, Samet JM. Estimating the risks and benefits of nicotine replacement therapy for smoking cessation in the United States; Am J Public Health. 2010 Feb;100(2):341-8

63. Winickoff JP, Buckley VJ, Palfrey JS, Perrin JM, Rigotti NA.Intervention with parental smokers in an outpatient pediatric clinic using counseling and nicotine replacement.Pediatrics. 2003 Nov; 112(5):1127-33

64. Roddy E, Romilly N, Challenger A, Lewis S, Britton J. Use socioeconomically deprived yof nicotine replacement therapy in young smokers: a communitybased pilot randomisedcontrolled trial; Tob Control. 2006 Oct; 15(5):373-6.

65. Abdullah AS, Hedley AJ, Chan SS, Ho WW. Establishment and evaluation of a smoking cessation clinic in Hong Kong: the a model for future service provider; J Public Health (Oxf). 2004 Sep; 26(3):239-44.

66. Varghese C, Kaur J, Desai N G, Murthy P, Malhotra S, Subbakrishna D K, et al. Initiating tobacco cessation services in India: challenges and opportunities WHO South-East Asia Journal of Public Health 2012;1(2):159-168.

67. Malcolm R, Currey HS, Mitchell MA, Keil JE. Silver Acetate Gum as a Deterrent to Smoking .Chest 1986; 90: 107-111.

68. Jensen EJ, Schmidt E, Pedersen B, Dahl R. Effect of nicotine, silver acetate, and ordinary chewing gum in combination with group counselling on smoking cessation. Thorax 1990; 45:831-834.

69. J Jarvis, Martin Raw, M A H Russell. C Feyerabend, Randomised controlled trial of nicotine chewing-gum; Br Med J (Clin Res Ed).1982 Aug 21; 285(6341):537-40.

70. Russell MA, Merriman R, Stapleton J, Taylor W. Effect of nicotine chewing gum as an adjunct to general practitioners' advice against smoking; British Medical Journal 1983; 287(6407):1782-5.

71. Jamrozik K, Fowler G, Vessey M, Wald N, et al. Placebo controlled trial of nicotine chewing gum in general practice; Br Med J (Clin Res Ed).1984 Sep 29; 289(6448):794-7.

72. Hjalmarson A, Effect of Nicotine Chewing Gum in Smoking Cessation: A Randomized Placebo-Controlled, Double-blind Study; JAMA. 1984 Nov 23- 30; 252(20):2835-8.

73. Leigh R, Viner NM, CoxG, Balon JW, Wilson DM, O'Shaughnessy D, et al. Nicotine replacement combined with a novel compound (ProBAN) for smoking cessation: a pilot study. Can Respir J 2001; 8(1):21-6.

74. Jessen AB, Toubro S, Astrup A. Effect of chewing gum containing nicotine and caffeine on energy expenditure and substrate utilization in men; Am J Clin Nutr. 2003 Jun; 77(6):1442-7.

75. Mochizuki M, Hatsugaya M, Rokujoh E, Arita E, Hashiguchi M, Shimizu N, et al. controlled study on the effectiveness of community pharmacists' advice for smoking cessation by Nicorette--evaluation at three months after initiation, Yakugaku Zasshi. 2004 Dec; 124(12):989-95

76. Oncken C, Dornelas E. Nicotine gum for pregnant smokers: a randomized controlled trial.; Obstet Gynecol. 2008 Oct;112(4):859-67

77. Christen A, Beiswanger B, Mau M, Walker C, Hatsukami D, Allen S, et al. Transdermal Nicotine for Smoking Cessation JAMA. 1991; 266(22):3133-3138.

78. Daughton DM, Heatley SA, Prendergast JJ, Causey D, Knowles M, Rolf CN, et al. Effect of Transdermal Nicotine Delivery as an Adjunct to Low-Intervention

Smoking Cessation Therapy A Randomized, Placebo-Controlled, Double-blind Study. Arch Intern Med 1991; 151(4):749-752.

79. Russell MA, Stapleton JA, Feyerabend C, Wiseman SM, Gustavsson G, Sawe U, et al. Targeting heavy smokers in general practice: randomised controlled trial of transdermal nicotine patches; BMJ 1993;306;1308-12.

80. Yudkin P L, Jones L, Lancaster T, Fowler G H. Which smokers are helped to give up smoking using transdermal nicotine patches? Results from a randomized, double-blind, placebo controlled trial. British Journal of General Practice 1996; 46:145-148.

81. Dale LC, Schroeder DR, Wolter TD, Croghan IT, Hurt RD, Offord KP.Weight change after smoking cessation using variable doses of transdermal nicotine replacement. J Gen Intern Med 1998; 13(1): 9-15.

82. Shaw JP, Ferry DG, Pethica D, Brenner D, Tucker IG. Usage patterns of transdermal nicotine when purchased as a non-prescription medicine from Pharmacies. Tobacco Control 1998; 7:161–167.

83. Benowitz NL, Zevin S, Jacob P 3rd. Suppression of Nicotine Intake During Ad Libitum Cigarette Smoking by High-Dose Transdermal Nicotine. JPET 1998; 287:958–962.

84. Otero UB, Perez Cde A, Szklo M, Esteves GA, dePinho MM, Szklo AS, et al. Randomized clinical trial: effectiveness of the cognitive-behavioral approach and the use of nicotine replacement transdermal patches for smoking cessation among adults in Riode Janeiro, Brazil; Cad Saude Publica. 2006 Feb; 22(2):439-49.

85. Hatsukami D, Mooney M, Murphy S, LeSage M, Babb D, Hecht S. Effects of high dose transdermal nicotine replacementin cigarette smokers; Pharmacol Biochem Behav. 2007 Jan; 86(1):132-9.

86. Ebbert JO, Post JA, Moyer TP, Dale LC, Schroeder DR, Hurt RD. Nicotine percentage replacement among smokeless tobacco users with nicotine patch; Drug Alcohol Depend. 2007 Jul 10;89(2-3):223-6.

87. David SP, Munafò MR, Murphy MF, Proctor M, Walton RT, Johnstone EC. Genetic variation in the dopamine D4 receptor (DRD4) gene and smoking cessation: follow-up of a randomised clinical trial of transdermal nicotine patch; Pharmacogenomics J. 2008 Apr; 8(2):122-8.

88. Glenn IM, Dallery J. Effects of internet-based voucher reinforcement and a transdermal nicotine patch on cigarette smoking; J Appl Behav Anal. 2007 Spring; 40(1):1-13.

89. Johnstone EC, Elliot KM, David SP, Murphy MF, Walton RT, Munafò MR. Association of COMT Val108/158 Met genotype with smoking cessation in a nicotine replacement therapy randomized trial; Cancer Epidemiol Biomarkers Prev. 2007 Jun;16(6):1065-9

90. Abu-Huwaij R, Obaidat RM, Sweidan K, Al-Hiari Y. Formulation and in vitro evaluation of xanthan gum or carbopol 934 based mucoadhesive patches, loaded with nicotine; AAPS PharmSciTech.2011 Mar;12(1):21-7.

91. Tang JL, Law M, Wald N. How effective is nicotine replacement therapy inhelping people to stop smoking? BMJ 1994; 308:21-6.

92. Cooney NL, Cooney JL. Smoking cessation during alcohol treatment: a randomized trial of combination nicotine patch plus nicotine gum; Addiction. 2009 Sep; 104(9):1588-96.

93. Russell MA, Jarvis MJ, Feyerabend C, Fernö O. Nasal nicotine solution:a potential aid to giving up smoking? BMJ 1983; 286: 683-684.

94. Tonnesen P, Nørregaard J, Mikkelsen K, Jorgensen S, Nilsson F. A Double-blind Trial of a Nicotine Inhaler for Smoking Cessation. JAMA 1993; 269:1268-1271.

95. Fagerström K O , Hughes J R , Rasmussen T, Callas P W. Randomised trial investigating effect of a novel nicotine delivery device(Eclipse) and a nicotine oral inhaler on smoking behaviour, nicotine and carbon monoxide exposure, and motivation to quit. Tobacco Control 2000; 9:327–333.

96. Bohadana A, Nilsson F, Rasmussen T, Martinet Y: Nicotine Inhaler and Nicotine Patch as a Combination Therapy for Smoking Cessation: A Randomized, Double-blind, Placebo-Controlled Trial. Arch Intern Med 2000; 160:3128-3134.

97. Hand S, Edwards S, Campbell IA, Cannings R. Controlled trial of three weeks nicotine replacement treatment in hospital patients also given advice and support; Thorax. 2002 Aug;57(8):715-8

98. Kralikova E, Kozak JT, Smoking cessation or reduction with nicotine replacement therapy: a placebo-controlled double blind trial with nicotine gum and inhaler; BMCPublic Health. 2009 Nov 27; 9:433

99. Hajek P, West R, Foulds J Nilsson F, Burrows S, Meadow A. Randomized Comparative Trial of Nicotine Polacrilex, a Transdermal Patch, Nasal Spray, and an Inhaler. Arch Intern Med 1999; 159:2033-2038.

100. Rubinstein ML, Benowitz NL, Auerback GM, Moscicki AB. A randomized trial of nicotine nasal spray in adolescent smokers; Pediatrics.2008 Sep; 122(3):e595-600

101. Rey L, Vaucher P, Secretan F, Zellweger JP, Bodenmann P. Use of nicotine substitute prescribed at hourly plus ad libitum intake or ad libitum for heavy smokers willing to quit: a randomized controlled trial; Subst Abuse Treat PrevPolicy. 2009 Jun 2;4:12

102. Shiffman S, Dresler CM, Hajek P, Gilburt SJ, Targett DA, Strahs KR. Efficacy of a nicotine lozenge for smoking cessation; Arch Intern Med2 002; 162(11):1267-76.

103. Ebbert JO, Edmonds A, Luo X, Jensen J, Hatsukami DK. Smokeless tobacco reduction with the nicotine lozenge and behavioral intervention; Nicotine Tob Res. 2010 Aug; 12(8):823-7.

104. Schnoll RA, Martinez E. Nicotine patch vs. nicotine lozenge for smoking cessation: an effectiveness trial coordinated by the Community Clinical Oncology Program; Drug Alcohol Depend. 2010 Mar 1; 107(2-3):237-43.

105. Wilson A, Sinfield P, Rodgers S, Hammersley V, Coleman T. Drugs to support smoking cessation in UK general practice: are evidence based guidelines being followed? Qual Saf Health Care. 2006 Aug; 15(4):284-8

106. Vogt F, Hall S, Marteau TM. General practitioners' beliefs about effectiveness and intentions to prescribe smoking cessation medications: qualitative and quantitative studies; BMC Public Health. 2006 Nov 8; 6:277.

107. Hurt RD, Sachs DP, Glover ED, Offord KP, Johnston JA, Dale LC, et al. A comparison of sustained-release bupropion and placebo For smoking cessation. N Engl J Med 1997; 337:1195-202.

108. Jorenby D.E., Leischow S.J. A controlled trial of sustained-release bupropion, a nicotine patch, or both for smoking cessation. N Engl J Med 1999; 340:685-91.

109. McEwen A, West R, Owen L. General Practitioners' views on the provision of nicotine replacement therapy and bupropion. BMC Fam Pract 2001; 2:6.

110. Antoñanzas F, Portillo F. Economic evaluation of pharmacotherapies for smoking cessation, Gac Sanit. 2003 Sep-Oct; 17(5):393-403.

111. Simon JA, Duncan C, Carmody TP, Hudes ES, Bupropion for smoking cessation: a randomized trial. Arch Intern Med. 2004 Sep 13; 164(16):1797-803.

112. Bolin K, Lindgren B, Willers S. The cost utility of bupropion in smoking cessation health programs: simulation model results for Sweden; Chest. 2006 Mar; 129(3):651-60.

113. Bertram MY, Lim SS, Wallace AL, Vos T. Costs and benefits of smoking cessation aids: making a case for public reimbursement of nicotine replacement therapy in Australia; Tob Control. 2007 Aug; 16(4):255-60.

114. Cupertino PA, Richter KP, Cox LS, Nazir N, Greiner AK, Ahluwalia JS, et al. Smoking cessation pharmacotherapy preferences in rural primary care; NicotineTob Res. 2008 Feb;10(2):301-7

115. Tidey JW, Rohsenow DJ. Intention to quit moderates the effect of bupropion on smoking urge; Nicotine Tob Res. 2009 Mar; 11(3):308-12.

116. McEwen A, West R. Do implementation issues influence the effectiveness of medications? The case of nicotine replacement therapy and bupropion in UK Stop Smoking Services; BMC Public Health. 2009 Jan 21; 9:28.

117. Al-Haj M. Bupropion as an aid for smoking cessation in the first year post marketing in Bradford (Zyban evaluation in Bradford (ZEBRA study). JRSM 2004 Dec; 11(2); 72-77.

118. Aubin HJ, Bobak A, Britton JR, Oncken C, Billing CB Jr, Gong J, Varenicline versus transdermal nicotine patch for smoking cessation: results from a randomized open-label trial; Thorax. 2008 Aug; 63(8):717-24.

119. Fernández de Bobadilla Osorio J, Sánchez-Maestre C, Brosa Riestra M, Arroyo O, Sanz de Burgoa V, Wilson K. Cost effectiveness analysis of varenicline (Champix) for the treatment of smoking in Spain; An Med Interna.2008 Jul; 25(7):342-8.

120. Moore TJ, Furberg CD, Glenmullen J, Maltsberger JT, Singh S. Suicidal behavior and depression in smoking cessation treatments; PLoS One. 2011; 6(11):e27016.

121. O'Malley SS, Cooney JL, Krishnan-Sarin S, Dubin JA, McKee SA, Cooney NL, et al. A controlled trial of naltrexone augmentation nicotine replacement therapy for smoking cessation; Arch Intern Med. 2006 Mar 27; 166(6):667-74.

122. Zatonski W, Cedzynska M, Tutka P, West R. An uncontrolled trial of cytisine (Tabex) for smoking cessation; Tob Control. 2006 Dec; 15(6):481-4.

123. Aveyard P, Johnson C, Fillingham S, Parsons A, Murphy M. Nortriptyline plus nicotine replacement versus placebo plus nicotine replacement for smoking cessation: pragmatic randomized controlled trial; BMJ. 2008 May 31; 336(7655):1223-7.

124. Epperson CN, Toll B, Wu R, Amin Z, Czarkowski KA, Jatlow P, Exploring the impact of gender and reproductive status on outcomes in a randomized clinical trial of naltrexone augmentation of nicotine patch; Drug Alcohol Depend. 2010 Nov 1; 112(1-2):1-8.

125. Prado GF, Lombardi EM. A real-life study of the effectiveness of different pharmacological approaches to the treatment of smoking cessation: re-discussing the predictors of success; Clinics (Sao Paulo). 2011;66(1):65-71.

126. Walker N, Howe C, Bullen C, McRobbie H, Glover M, Parag V, et al. Study protocol for a non inferiority trial of cytosine versus nicotine replacement therapy in people motivated to stop smoking.; BMC Public Health. 2011 Nov 21;11:880.

127. Ravichand M.D.,Vijaya N. The pharmacotherapy of smoking cessation.Calicut Medical Journal 2007;5(1):e2

128. Moore D, Aveyard P, Connock M, Wang D, Fry-Smith A, Barton P. Effectiveness and safety of nicotine replacement therapy assisted reduction to stop smoking: systematic review and meta-analysis. BMJ. 2009 Apr 2; 338:b1024.

129. Eliasson B, Taskinen M, Smith Ulf. Long-term Use of Nicotine Gum Is Associated With Hyperinsulinemia and Insulin Resistance. Circulation 1996; 94:878-881.

130. Pullon S, Webster M, McLeod D, Benn C, Morgan S.Smoking cessation and nicotine replacement therapy in current primary maternity care, Aust Fam Physician. 2004 Jan-Feb;33(1-2):94-6.

131. Shiffman S, Burton SL, Pillitteri JL. Test of "Light" cigarette counter-advertising using a standard test of advertising effectiveness. Tob Control 2001; 10 Suppl 1: i33-40.

132. West R, Zhou X. Is nicotine replacement therapy for smoking cessation effective in the"real world"? Findings from a prospective multinationa lcohort study; Thorax. 2007 Nov; 62(11):998-1002.

FSC
www.fsc.org
MIX
Papier | Fördert gute Waldnutzung
FSC® C083411

Kolibri 360 GmbH
Ferdinand-Jühlke-Straße 7
99095 Erfurt, Deutschland
produktsicherheit@kolibri360.de

Druck:
CPI Druckdienstleistungen GmbH
im Auftrag der
Kolibri 360 GmbH
Ferdinand-Jühlke-Str. 7
99095 Erfurt